# CLIMATE CHAOS

# CLIMATE CHAOS

## *Your Health at Risk*

## What You Can Do to
## Protect Yourself and Your Family

### Cindy L. Parker, MD, MPH
### and Steven M. Shapiro, PhD

Public Health

Lawrence J. Cheskin, Series Editor

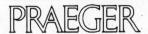

**Westport, Connecticut
London**

This book was made with recycled chlorine-free paper. For more information, please visit www.chlorinefreeproducts.org.

Library of Congress Cataloging-in-Publication Data

Parker, Cindy L., 1959-
  Climate chaos : your health at risk : what you can do to protect yourself and your family / Cindy L. Parker and Steven M. Shapiro.
      p. cm. — (Public health ISSN 1942-8812)
  Includes bibliographical references and index.
  ISBN: 978-0-275-99858-5 (alk. paper)
  1. Climatic changes—Health aspects—Popular works. 2. Medical climatology—Popular works. I. Shapiro, Steven M., 1959- II. Title.
  RA793.P32 2008
  616.9'88—dc22      2008016469

British Library Cataloguing in Publication Data is available.

Library of Congress Catalog Card Number: 2008016469
ISBN: 978-0-275-99858-5
ISSN: 1942-8812

First published in 2008

Praeger Publishers, 88 Post Road West, Westport, CT 06881
An imprint of Greenwood Publishing Group, Inc.
www.praeger.com

Printed in the United States of America

The paper used in this book complies with the Permanent Paper Standard issued by the National Information Standards Organization (Z39.48-1984).

10 9 8 7 6 5 4 3 2 1

# Contents

# Series Foreword

Extreme weather events have been a hallmark of the new millennium: hurricanes, storms, floods, droughts. What is happening to our climate has become such an important global worry of late because, at this point, it is undeniable that the changes are real (as anyone who reads, or who notices the weather, can tell, and as the 10 years ending in 2007 were the warmest on record). Most sobering, it's clear that global warming is in large part directly caused by human activities, and it's creating enormous concern for the public's health.

*Climate Chaos*, by Cindy Parker, MD, and Steve Shapiro, PhD, helps you to understand the science of global warming and the likely health consequences if the problem is not aggressively addressed soon; at the same time, the book provides practical advice on what you can do to protect yourself, your loved ones, and your world.

The authors are experts at Johns Hopkins University in the medical and behavioral consequences of climate change. They offer insights into the personal, societal, and planetary toll that will likely result from continuing our current course of inaction in the face of the growing threat of climate chaos.

Most important, the authors offer a practical blueprint for action, for both individuals and institutions. Indeed, there is a lot that we—as individuals, communities, states, and nations—can and should be doing right now. As the authors convincingly demonstrate in these pages, the health of every living creature on this planet is at stake.

Despite its sobering message, this book is easy and enjoyable to read. In each chapter, a fictional family's story highlights the relevance of the content to people's lives. In addition, there is a solutions section at the end of each chapter that explains what actions you can take to play a role in preventing the harm of climate change. The book ends with a best-case scenario that illustrates the way things can be if we change our behavior to effect change in our future.

With the help of each reader, may we make the "best-case scenario" a reality and avert the most serious damage to us and our only planet home.

Lawrence J. Cheskin, MD, FACP
Series Editor

# Chapter 1

# A Climate Change Tale

Maria knows this isn't any ordinary day. None of the days have been normal recently, what with the temperature soaring into the low 100s for the past two weeks, and her son Zacharias complaining as never before about the heat, about his difficulty breathing in it. It has also been blazingly dry recently, with none of the usual afternoon rains to cool the air. So Maria dresses her son and his little sister Keisha in lightweight clothes, knowing that their year-round school isn't adequately air conditioned and will be sweltering by noon if the predictions are right: 112°F (44°C) at midday. This is the fourth major heat wave of early summer, Maria says to herself, tabulating them in her mind, and every year has seemed to set new records.

She feeds the kids breakfast—their usual bowl of sweet cereal, even though it costs three times as much as it did just a year ago—as their father Moravia calls out as he sweeps into the kitchen, "Maria, I just looked outside, and there's something wrong with the air today, too. So it's not just the blasted heat. Keep an eye out for what's going on, for Zach, yes?" He kisses his wife on the forehead, brushes the cheeks of his two children with his slender fingers, and leaves for the long drive to work at his office 45 miles away.

As Maria drives her children to the bus stop four blocks from home and waits with them for a few minutes, the temperature now only in the low 90s, she notes that there is something odd about the air: it's a thick gray and stings her lungs. Of course the windows are rolled up, and the air conditioning is on, while the engine idles, but it never seems to help much. She asks Zach whether he's breathing OK, and he nods yes. Keisha, though, looks uneasy.

It's only after the kids get on the bus and she returns home to finish getting ready for work that she hears the warnings on the radio: another Code Black day for ozone, the third one this month. She remembers back when Zach was just a baby and the Code Red days were the most severe. How she had worried about Zach's breathing on those days! Then when Zach was about four, the authorities had increased the top of the scale to purple, and those Code Purple days seemed to get more and more common. Then, earlier this summer, they had announced Code Black days for the first time—days on which it was unsafe for *anyone* to be outside for more than just a few minutes, and when people were encouraged to hold their breath as much as possible as they transferred from their cars to their homes, schools, offices, and shops. So far there had been only six Code Black days this summer, but three had occurred in the first two weeks of this month. During the last one, Maria had to double Zach's breathing medicine and had seriously considered increasing the dose even more. She knows it isn't good for him to be taking all that medicine, but she can't stand watching him work so hard to breathe.

Maria finishes dressing in a hurry and goes to get the extra medicine for Zach, which she'll drop off at school on her way to work. She knows the school won't be surprised to see her. With 70 percent of the children there suffering from asthma, a lot of parents are bringing extra medicine to school these days.

Then the phone rings. Maria's brother Max is on the line. She hasn't talked with him for a few days, and his voice sounds edgy as he tells her to sit down, that he has something "terribly important" to tell her. Maria, trying to sound amused given her own unease this morning, says she has no time to talk now. She can't be late to morning rounds at the hospital, where she attends to the older patients in the Wise Elders Geriatric Unit. No matter how hard it tries, the hospital still hasn't figured out a way to keep all the outside air out. With another Code Black day, many of her patients will be having more trouble breathing, and she knows she needs to brace herself for another round of heart attacks . . . like what happened last time, just a few days ago. She lost three of her patients during that episode, and two weren't even that old—barely 70. But they're always the ones to suffer the most from these strange weather extremes—the children and the elderly, she thinks. It's just not fair!

The urgency in Max's voice brings her out of her reverie. He sounds more serious than she can remember, so she sits down. And Max blows her away: he wants to bring his entire family—wife, four children, three dogs, two cats, and a parakeet—to live with her and her family. In three, maybe four, days, depending on the drive time. Get ready.

Maria, stunned, incredulous, uncertain, laughs: "Don't joke with me like that, Max. That's not funny."

"I'm not kidding," Max responds. His voice is flat, now. "You haven't heard, have you?"

"Heard what?" Maria asks, her stomach suddenly hurting. She remembers her stomach would sometimes hurt when she was a child, when she was afraid of all the sorts of things young children fear. She is feeling very afraid now.

"The storm. The hurricane," Max says. "It's nothing yet, just Category 3, but it could be a Category 6 in two days and maybe even a 7. It could hit us. Again. They're not sure yet, but they're thinking . . . they're saying it's bigger than Raquel. And you know what she did to us last year . . . after Nick and Opal. Back to back to back. Bam, bam, bam. We don't even have our roof totally back on yet. The blue tarps are still up there. And the cracks in the foundation. And the broken patio doors, and broken windows, and . . ." His voice trails off, and Maria knows it's all too real. She begins to tap the table with the pinky and thumb of her right hand, a habit she's developed recently but can't seem to control.

"We're not staying on the coast anymore," he says, sounding almost numb. "I'm quitting my job today, Maria. So is Sula. We'll reestablish ourselves there, with you. We can do that easily enough. We'll put the kids in that year-round school with Zach and Keisha. We're bringing as much as we can in our SUVs and the trailer."

Maria's thoughts are whirling. She's amazed to hear that Max is finally giving up, leaving his beloved coast. The beautiful beaches—or at least what's left of them after years of increasingly destructive hurricanes and relentless sea level rise; the bluffs above the seas with their wonderful vistas, where he would walk for hours—although they, too, have been pummeled into a treeless oblivion in many places; and the soothing blue-green waters in which he loved to swim to clear his mind, even when the waters were chilled in the cooler months that didn't seem so cool anymore.

Max, a successful stockbroker, had built his family's palatial home just back from the shoreline 15 years ago, and Maria knows that that line has been relentlessly creeping closer to his house with each passing year. It was only last year, though, when sea level rise coupled with a brutal spate of hurricanes, unparalleled in modern history, that the house seemed to be approaching some sort of abyss. And so, too, is Max. She has heard it in his voice every time she's talked with him recently. They had been close as children, and Max always seemed unflappable then. He was the one who led her and their siblings Magda and Arnie on long forays into the dark, seemingly dangerous forest near their parents' home in the Midwest. He was the one who proposed wild activities, like riding their bikes down a nearby hill, steeper than a ski slope, or bouncing and swinging on ropes from tree limb to tree limb 10 feet off the ground in their backyard like some sort of squirrel. Max is sounding anything but certain now, though.

"You know, Max," Maria hears herself saying in a dubious, quietly imploring tone of voice, "Magda and her kids just moved out a month ago."

"I know; I know," says Max. "I'm sorry to do this to you now. It's just . . . we've got no one else to turn to right now, and there's no hope for the house anymore. One more blast, one more major storm . . . . We're only 20 feet from the water now, even with the wall. And I know this is going to be the storm, Maria. I can feel it in my bones."

Ah, the wall, Maria thinks, shaking her head. Max and Sula spent more than $100,000 on that containment wall nearly a decade ago and tens of thousands more to keep it from being totally swept into the sea as the storms worsened year by year. The wall actually spilled major portions of itself into the rising, raging seas and had to be rebuilt repeatedly after each hurricane swept in with its devastating fury. As such, it had to be reconstructed closer and closer to the house, where there still was some land to tie it to. That land between the sea and the house, though, is about gone now. Max knows it is time for his family to give up, especially with Hurricane Carl building strength.

There is silence on the cell phone. While Max is thinking about how the changing climate is turning around his and his family's life forever, Maria is thinking about the life of her family, too. She is more than worried about her kids. They haven't been as healthy lately. Zach, mostly, has been having worse breathing problems, fevers, and aches and pains more and more. Moravia, too, seems to be suffering as never before. He is more irritable, and he complains daily about the long drive to work, his perpetual headache, the ridiculous cost of synfuel—what with all the taxes now applied to each gallon to reduce consumption and pay for technology projects aimed at fuel efficiency and cleaning the air. And she notices that her elderly patients are coming to her office and the hospital with more breathing and heart ailments; more stress from the rising costs of food, fuel, and utilities and worry about the strange weather; and more expressions of just general doubt and hopelessness. Some aren't recovering from their illnesses as fast as they used to. Some are even dying too young . . . .

And then, she thinks, she has been having an odd feeling of foreboding, as though something really bad is just beyond her vision. Maria has been through a lot in her life, but only in the past few years has she noticed it wearing poorly on her. Most recently, that strain came from the 18 months that Magda and her three kids crammed themselves into her home in the heartland. As nice as it was to have her sister close, it also was exhausting. To have her sister and her sister's three young children in her own home, where she could do so little to comfort them in their time of need . . . .

Magda, she remembers, called one day from her home in the mountains to say there was no more water. Maria knew that the water shortages were severe; she just didn't know they'd become so bad. Magda had moved to the Southwest long ago, just after she became a teacher, to get away from the uniformity, what she called "the quiet tedium," of the plains. She was always looking for something larger than life in the hinterland, and she had found it in the beautiful southwestern deserts. She also found her husband Rick there, also a teacher, and they had had three beautiful children—two girls and a boy—before Magda and her family felt forced to move into the Rockies when the desert temperatures began to soar ever higher, and the rains stopped falling, and the water became scarce. Yes, trucks hauling thousands of gallons of water for hundreds of miles brought water to the ever-burgeoning city, but life was getting harder and harder there despite efforts to deal with climate change. They felt that to raise a family without disruption to their way of life meant they had no choice but to move out of the desert, so they had moved to the mountains.

At first, life in the mountains was better. Enough snow fell in the winter to keep the water flowing the rest of the year, although the aquifers were dropping precipitously low, and cities and towns throughout the mountain states were beginning to restrict water use. But then, the snowpack in the winter months had become less and less, and the water and other utility restrictions had become more oppressive, and people had begun to look for other places in which their families could survive. Magda found, as the stresses of life in the mountains became more pervasive, that she was not getting Rick's support. He was becoming more distant, less involved as a parent and husband. And one day he suddenly said he didn't want to be part of the family anymore. He left that night. Magda thought maybe he had a girlfriend—someone younger, thinner, more energetic than she. But they found his body the next morning along with a suicide note.

That was when Magda had called Maria. She had called crying, not only for her husband, but also because she knew that her foray into the deserts and mountains was coming to an end. The mountains were still beautiful, but the world there truly was changing. Most of her friends had already left. The price of water was just too high. Magda knew that there was no way she'd be able to buy water with only her salary. Hadn't it already been a struggle with both salaries? Weren't they already in debt up to their ears? She thought about her options. She had a friend on the West Coast who had invited her to come out, but she'd heard on the news that the dust blowing across the Pacific Ocean from China was causing terrible dust storms that reached all the way into Kansas. Often the air on the coast was so gritty that it tore at people's throats and burned their eyes as they covered their mouths and noses with cloths to keep the dust out of their lungs. Water woes, wild temperature fluctuations, and strange storms had also become the norm in the West. That certainly didn't sound appealing. It also seemed to Magda that the East Coast and Gulf Coast had nearly constant problems with flooding from the rising oceans and hurricanes. No, the only escape was back to the Midwest where she'd grown up. They'd had more and more devastating tornadoes and storms there recently, but she'd grown up with tornadoes. She knew what to do with tornadoes.

Maria is thinking about that call from Magda now. She recalls how Magda and her three children arrived with so little, mostly just their clothes and a few beloved toys and trinkets, and moved themselves in. For 18 months. She can see her nieces and nephew talking quietly among themselves all the time, their eyes teary. She hears them talking about how in the mountains they'd often been dirty and had believed they were thirsty "all the time," and how the land around them had seemed to die before their very eyes week after week. The beetle infestations that had killed the pines. The droughts that actually had torn the land apart. The empty lakes and streams that had once been filled with fish and had attracted birds and big game. The people wearily gazing at these mountain losses as they themselves seemed to slip away day after day, leaving behind a burgeoning suburban ghost town. All because throughout the West the water had stopped coming. Maybe it was just . . . the way their father had left, had died, Maria wondered. Magda had assured Maria over and over that "it wasn't as bad as all that." No?

Maria recalls how her children and Magda's argued a lot, how crowded her home felt with four new people there. She remembers how everyone was on edge as they had learned to live with one another; find spaces for themselves in a newly blended family; wondered what would become of them in the next day, week, month . . . . That wasn't something Maria had ever expected for herself or her family. Never.

And then one day Magda had said she was feeling strong enough as a single parent on a teacher's salary. She had paid off some of her debts and had managed to save a little money. She moved with her kids to an apartment just a mile from Maria's home and left Maria and her family suddenly alone with one another again, back where they had been a year and a half before. Except they weren't back where they had been, were they? The water shortages that had hit the Western states with such force were suddenly at their doorstep in the Midwest. And the heat. And the sickening air quality. And the strange, dangerous weather patterns . . .

And now, to make it all seem so much more than worse, Max is coming with his family. The pets, too.

"Max, I don't know if I can . . ." Her words trail off. She can't finish the sentence. She knows he wouldn't be coming if he had any other options. "What about Arnie? Maybe you could stay with Arnie until . . . ?" Max doesn't answer. She can hear him breathing, labored, scared. Maria knows it's a lame suggestion, that she is grasping for answers that won't come. Arnie would be even less able than Maria to cope with Max's family. Arnie has always been quiet, even when they were kids. He was the most sensitive of them. She thinks about how he took the horrible news. The news that had begun to trickle out, then flow ever more rapidly, more than 10 years ago.

The media reports had shown grisly pictures of so many people dying in Bangladesh, as they kept losing precious cropland to the rising sea levels. People had watched with horror as storm after storm wrought more and more damage on already-fragile coastlines in Asia, Africa, and island nations around the world. The death tolls kept climbing. In Africa, diseases that had long been in check were killing children, the elderly, and the poor as never before. Some days, on any given day, there were reports that tens of thousands more had died here and there. Maria had often wondered then how it was possible that so many people could die every day without some enormous cataclysm to fell them, but the growing spate of disasters seemed to never run out of people to kill. There had been famines throughout Africa and in much of Asia. Coups, wars, and genocide—all related to the changing climate around the planet—became common, and the violence just kept getting worse. There wasn't enough food or water, there wasn't enough land, there weren't enough trees for fuel, and people living on $2 a day certainly couldn't afford to buy synfuel to cook their food.

But the violence on the television wasn't beamed only from places on the other side of the world. In the United States, terrorists had begun to attack a new place every month. New York, maybe unsurprisingly, was first, with a series of car and truck bombs that had killed more than 100 people and maimed hundreds more. That was already too close to home, and it was so terrifying that Arnie couldn't sleep for days. He had kept vigil near his big picture window, an eye on the television and the other peering past the curtains to the quiet street outside, a street more than 100 miles from the Big City. But then the terrorist bombings, some random shootings, and attempts to release toxic chemicals had spread: Miami, San Francisco, Dallas, Billings. Billings! Maria couldn't understand then why the rest of the world was blaming America for what was happening to the climate everywhere on the planet. Wasn't everyone just going about their business, trying to make life as normal as it had always been, buying nice things for their children, having a little fun? How could that be bad?

After the initial shock of the terrorist attacks had subsided, Arnie just stared at the TV, unable to take his eyes off the devastation and the miserable faces of the survivors. First he had stopped cooking, and then he had stopped going to bed. He just sat all night in his easy chair, watching the news, dozing off and on, drinking beer. He would sometimes drag himself into his studio to paint the paintings that once sustained him and connected him with the art community in which he had thrived, but his love of creation was waning fast. His life was waning fast.

Now, a decade later, Maria thinks about how she managed to save Arnie from total collapse. She flew to his vast, rangy home in the Berkshires that he bought when he was near the top of the New York art scene, took charge of his affairs, and got him started on an antidepressant medication. It took the edge off, even if Arnie still wasn't the creative force he used to be. Then she helped him find work teaching art at the local community college. It paid the bills, even if the job seemed to further diminish Arnie's creative flow. And, finally, she put his affairs in order and connected him with some support so she wouldn't have to babysit her grown little brother and give up on her own new career in medicine. Even if it left Arnie wondering whether he could ever be the person he once was.

What am I thinking? Maria now laughs uneasily to herself, shaking her head to forget the images of death and destruction that nearly brought Arnie to his knees all those years ago. The images have remained, though, and they have gotten even worse with this crazy climate chaos, and Arnie is never going to be in any shape to do anything but barely subsist with them. Max and his family at Arnie's! His house sure is large enough, but it's still a mess. An artist's lair. A poor artist's lair, at that. His heart's in the right place, although you wouldn't know it by spending time with him. And his life . . . well, his life is a near shambles. It would be difficult for someone as ordered and clear-headed as Max to survive in that setting without a major struggle.

And isn't Max already in that struggle? No, Max and his family have no other choice, Maria thinks, but to come here. At least for a while.

"Max," Maria hears herself saying, as though it isn't really her. "Max. OK. What can I say? We don't have the biggest house in the world. And you know we've tried to cut back a little to not use so much energy, so much space. It'll be tight. It'll be . . ."

"Maria," Max says, quieter than she's ever heard his voice. "Thank you."

But the worries flood her voice. "Max, the air here is getting worse. My kids can't breathe. Your kids could have problems. . . and the heat, Max, it's so hot here now. And we're beginning to wonder about how long the water's going to hold up. There's so much we've got to face. So much. Do you really want to see this here, with your family?" Maria feels almost embarrassed. She can hear it in her own voice.

"Maria," Max intones. "We're better off with you, I'm telling you. Even with what you're facing now, because this Earth's gone mad. We have no choice."

And Maria, hanging her head, wonders how this can be true. How the only world we have has come to this.

# Chapter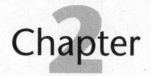

## Climate Chaos:
## What May Come

With Zach finally asleep, after three hits from his inhaler stemmed his latest asthma attack, Maria begins to get the house in order for Max and his family's arrival in three or so days. She had wanted to take Zach to the ER again because his breathing had become so labored, but he finally persuaded her that he was feeling better and just needed to rest.

She heads for the house's small den, wondering how much worse it can get for Zach, to clean out piles of paperwork and other junk there because Max's kids will have to sleep for now on its pull-out sofa and on the floor. As she clears off a shelf of books that will have to serve as her nieces and nephews' clothing area, she finds wedged between a bunch of big tomes a red spiral-bound book that she hasn't seen in years.

Maria glances at the cover of the book and her heart skips a beat. *Climate Change and Health*, the title of the book reads in bright red letters on a sky-blue background. The subtitle says *A Guide for Early-Career Health Professionals to Prepare for a Warming World*.

Maria sits down on the sofa, drapes her dust rag over her shoulder, and cautiously opens the book. She vaguely remembers the course she had to take in medical school that included this topic. It seemed so uncertain back then, she thinks, didn't it? But now. . . .

Maria flips from chapter to chapter in the slender book. A prediction starts each brief chapter: "As the climate warms, there will be more and more-severe weather-related events—including hurricanes, tornadoes, and massive storms—around the world." "Sea level rise will drown some small-island nations and coastal areas that will displace thousands upon thousands of people and increase their poverty, lack of access to adequate food and clean water, and, ultimately, the misery of their lives." "Some places will face droughts that will damage crops needed to feed the world. Other places will endure excessive rain and flooding that will harm the flora and fauna for the foreseeable future." "Diseases and illnesses will become more prevalent and persistent, ranging from increased heat-related illnesses, vector-borne diseases like malaria, respiratory ailments such as asthma, and much, much more."

Tears fill Maria's eyes. "I should have listened then," she says to herself. "We all should have listened—should have done more—when they first noticed this global warming coming."

## WHAT THIS BOOK IS ABOUT

This book is about listening, learning, and striving for changes in our behavior right now to prevent the potential ill effects of climate change on our health and the health of our one and only planet, the place that sustains the wellness of its denizens if, and only if, we take care of it. The story about Maria and her family that you have read so far is fiction, yes, but everything portrayed in their lives is scientifically plausible—even likely— in the near future if we continue to conduct ourselves with our "business as usual" mentality. That means the rising amount of greenhouse gases our cars, power plants, and factories spew into our atmosphere will continue to contribute to rising temperatures around the globe with dire consequences for most everyone eventually. Even those who believe it's mostly a problem for people far away and in the distant future; who believe they have the resources to cool off by simply turning up their air conditioning; or who believe they can avoid the worst by just ignoring what's coming will still be susceptible to the consequences of climate change.

Before we delve into the details of how climate change will harm us, we would like to give you an overview of what underlies climate change, how it's relevant to the health of every human and the planet, and how we've structured the book. We also want you to know, from the outset, that while climate change, which is also known as global warming, may seem overwhelming or too distant to matter now, there is a lot that we— as individuals, communities, states, and nations—can and should be doing immediately to reduce it. If we do too little too late, it's not just a few degrees of temperature rise that we'll all be feeling in a few years. This onrushing climate chaos will put the health of every living creature on this planet up for grabs. And that includes you, your children, every living thing. . . .

## WHAT'S HAPPENING TO OUR CLIMATE

Extreme weather events and their harmful impact on human health have been a hallmark of the new millennium. There have been plenty of weather disasters all over the world, including right here in the United States, where:

- Hurricane Katrina in 2005 took more than 1,800 lives in the Gulf Coast and New Orleans and caused a record $125 billion in damage and cleanup costs.
- During a 14-month period in 2004 and 2005, eight hurricanes made landfall in Florida, causing flooding, power outages, wind damage, injuries, and deaths.
- A record 400 tornadoes were recorded in the Midwest in one week in 2003, and severe storms and hail caused deaths and massive crop losses in the southern plains and the Mississippi valley.
- Later that year, Hurricane Isabel caused $5 billion of damage from North Carolina to New York and was responsible for 55 deaths.
- In 2002, droughts and heat waves sparked fires throughout the West that claimed at least 21 lives.
- And at least 43 deaths were reported during the flooding in Texas and Louisiana that resulted from tropical storm Allison in 2001.

That's not all. Widespread, severe drought has plagued the Southwest and Great Plains for several years. The Southeast experienced the worst drought in recorded history in 2007, seriously threatening Atlanta's water supply. Meanwhile, Georgia, Tennessee, and North Carolina instituted water restrictions, as have many jurisdictions in the Mid-Atlantic states, because of severe drought. Drought also provoked wildfires in California, displacing half a million people and destroying more than a thousand homes. And tornadoes struck at an unmatched pace in October 2007, with a record 87 twisters forming in just one three-day span, surpassing the previous record of 63 in a three-day span.

Every year in the United States and around the world, thousands of people die, are injured, and lose their homes and their livelihoods because of these extreme weather events. Unfortunately, global warming is going to make these events more frequent and more severe, meaning our health and well-being will be at ever-increasing risk.[1]

Before August 2005, many Americans thought that major "natural" disasters that harm and displace hundreds or thousands of people only happen in other, usually developing, countries. Somehow, many of us believed our wealth and advanced development would prevent devastation from occurring here. Hurricane Katrina changed that perception as Americans watched their television screens in horror as the disaster unfolded. Apart from the terrible scenes of death and destruction, many thousands were displaced. Maybe even more shocking, more than two years after the storm—in the richest, most influential country in the world—New Orleans and much of the Gulf Coast remained devastated. The day-to-day functioning of the Gulf Coast has been severely compromised, and the Gulf Coast residents' health has suffered as a direct consequence.

Climate change clearly is a huge problem for our physical and mental health, and it can seem overwhelming. Let's start with the basics—the difference between weather and climate. Weather refers to what's happening outside right now, what happened in the recent past, or what we can expect in the near future. We listen to the weather report to find out if rain is expected or what the high temperatures might be for that day or the next. Weather can only be accurately predicted for a relatively few days. Climate, on the other hand, describes long-term trends in the weather. What the weather has been like in a particular area for the past several decades, or even centuries, is the climate of that area. We might choose certain regions of the country or the world to spend our vacations based on their climate. What we encounter when we get there, however, is the weather. The list of recent extreme weather events we just described tells us only what kind of weather occurred in those places on those days. If we look at the total weather record over decades or centuries, that will tell us what the climate was like—and the climate, all over the world, has been slowly changing.

It turns out that the 10 years ending in 2007 were the warmest on record. In fact, every recent decade has been warmer than the previous one.[2] During the past century, the average temperature of Earth's surface has risen about 1.4°F (0.8°C), but as you can see in Figure 2.1, most of that increase occurred in the past 30 years.[3]

## WHY THE CLIMATE IS CHANGING

Those warming temperatures are driving our Earth's climate. We'll explain why we're warming in a moment. For now, know that as average global temperatures increase, the patterns of wind, ocean currents, and rainfall on the planet will change and bring more frequent and severe heat waves, hurricanes, and thunderstorms.[1] The climate that we've come to expect for the past several generations will become less stable, less predictable, and more chaotic.

Some of that chaos comes from warmer air holding more moisture. This means we can expect more rain as global warming changes the climate. Warmer air temperatures, however, also encourage more evaporation of moisture from the soil. So currently dry areas will tend to get drier, and wet areas will get wetter.

That generalization, however, belies the regional variability that actually affects people's lives and livelihoods. More of the annual rainfall will appear as heavy rainstorms that are more likely to cause flooding. In between these heavy rains there will be longer stretches of drought. These trends are likely to occur in North America as well as globally. In central India, for example, the overall rainfall is not expected to change, but more of that rain will fall during severe rainstorms, causing more deadly flooding.[4]

Another problem: warmer temperatures mean more annual precipitation will fall as rain instead of snow, reducing snowpack in some regions that is vital for water availability during the late spring and summer months when plants require more water for growth.

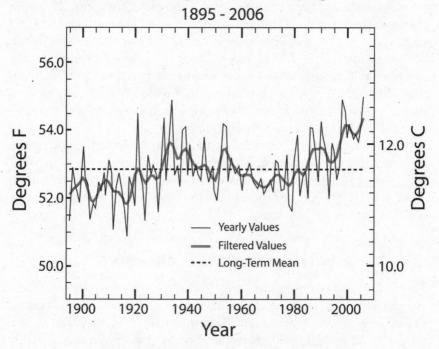

**National (Contiguous U.S.) Temperature**
1895 - 2006

National Climatic Data Center / NESDIS / NOAA

Figure 2.1

## THE GREENHOUSE EFFECT

These climatic changes in precipitation and storms result from a process that begins with the Sun's energy shining through our Earth's atmosphere and warming its surface. But not all of the Sun's energy stays put on the surface; some of it is reflected back into space and doesn't help to warm Earth's surface. Fortunately for us, there are greenhouse gases forming a sort of protective blanket in the atmosphere that helps to hold the Sun's energy here on the surface and keep us warm enough to survive.

You've likely heard complaints about climate change resulting from too many greenhouse gases. That's true, too. The reason is that if there weren't any greenhouse gases in the atmosphere, most of the Sun's energy would leak back into space, and the surface of the Earth would be about 60°F (33°C) colder than it is now.[5] So greenhouse gases are a good thing—up to a point. Because the concentration of greenhouse gases in our atmosphere has now gotten too thick and dense, they're holding in too much of the Sun's energy and warming the surface of Earth too much. It's like what happens in a greenhouse or in a car in the summertime. If you have a car with a convertible roof and the roof is down, the temperature in the car is the same as outside. If the roof and windows are up, though, the Sun's energy can get into the car, but it can't get out as easily and the inside gets cooking.

The main greenhouse gas is carbon dioxide, or $CO_2$. Other greenhouse gases that are also causing climate problems are methane, nitrous oxide, and tiny quantities of other chemicals that we'll talk about later. $CO_2$ is produced whenever fossil fuels, such as coal, oil, gasoline, or natural gas, are burned to get energy to heat or cool our homes, run our businesses and industries, power our cars, and make electricity.

A vicious cycle develops as $CO_2$ warms Earth's atmosphere, which then absorbs and holds more water vapor that, in turn, contributes to more warming. This is sometimes called a positive feedback loop, and we'll talk about its role later in the book. We'll also explore more about methane, which is mostly produced from agricultural activities such as raising livestock, in the chapter about food.

## GREENHOUSE GASES AND TEMPERATURE

You may be wondering how we know that the concentrations of greenhouse gases in the atmosphere are increasing and warming our planet, given that this requires knowledge of those gases and temperatures dating back thousands of years. Scientists developed this knowledge by understanding that as the snow falls in Antarctica, the weight of the newer snow compresses the layers below into ice, trapping bubbles of air. Scientists have successfully drilled down about two miles through the ice and removed a solid core of it. They have been analyzing the tiny amounts of air trapped in the ice. Each of those tiny pockets of air is a small sample of what was in our atmosphere at that time, including the concentrations of $CO_2$, nitrogen oxides, sulfur dioxide, soot (sometimes called black carbon), oxygen, and any other chemicals present in the air then. The ice at the bottom of that 2-mile core is almost 1 million years old.[6]

As for determining the temperature at the time the ice was formed, it turns out that oxygen changes its chemical properties slightly depending on the temperature. So even though prehistoric peoples didn't have thermometers, scientists can analyze the oxygen trapped in the ice pockets and get an accurate idea of the temperature when those ice crystals formed.[6]

More recently, temperature readings have been taken in a variety of weather stations around Earth since the mid-1800s, and $CO_2$ levels in the atmosphere have been faithfully measured since 1958 on top of Mauna Loa in Hawaii. By putting this recent information together with what we've learned from the ice cores, we now know that during the past million years at least, the levels of $CO_2$ in the atmosphere were never higher than about 280 parts per million (ppm) until the start of the Industrial Revolution about 200 years ago. In 1958, the level was only 315 ppm, but now it's more than 380 ppm.[7] See Figure 2.2.

Figuring out how much $CO_2$ was in the atmosphere hundreds of thousands of years ago and what the corresponding temperatures were is very helpful for recognizing how much of a problem we have now. What would be even more helpful, however, would be to know how much global warming we can expect in the future and what kinds of consequences that might have for the world. Because no one has a crystal ball, scientists use huge super-computers to study all the possibilities and project the likely scenarios.

These computer models are tested by having them run their calculations as if they were starting in the distant past and comparing the results to what we know were the actual climates and temperatures of the time. Once the computers' results match our knowledge of the past, then the models are used to project the likely climate in the future. Using this method and many other ways of verifying the projections, scientists can fairly accurately project a range of what our climate will likely look like by 2100 and beyond. As more data become available from thousands of scientific studies taking place all over the world, the models continue to get more accurate and can provide more information about what we can expect. What the computers and the scientists project, if we continue with "business as usual," is that:

# Temperature and $CO_2$ levels for past 400,000 years

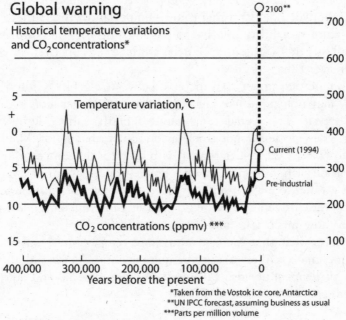

## Global warning

Historical temperature variations
and $CO_2$ concentrations*

Temperature variation, °C

$CO_2$ concentrations (ppmv) ***

2100**

700
600
500
400
Current (1994)
300
Pre-industrial
200
100

5
+
0
−
5
10
15

400,000    300,000    200,000    100,000          0
Years before the present

*Taken from the Vostok ice core, Antarctica
**UN IPCC forecast, assuming business as usual
***Parts per million volume

Source: CDIAC Oak Ridge National Laboratory

**Figure 2.2** This graph shows the $CO_2$ levels from 400,000 years ago to present and temperatures from the same time period showing how closely the temperature follows the $CO_2$ level.

- The *average* surface temperature of Earth will increase between 2°F and 11.5°F (1.1°C to 6.4°C) by the year 2100.
- The sea level will rise 7 to 23 inches (18 to 58 cm).
- And there will be a marked increase in weather extremes.[1] (You will soon learn that these numbers may be understated!)

Let's take a closer look at what these projections really mean. First, *averages* can be deceiving. For example, if your travel agent planned a trip for you to the moon and told you that the average surface temperature of the moon is about 0°F (−18°C), you would pack a good coat to keep warm. When you arrive on the moon's surface, however, to find that the dark side has a temperature of −250°F (−157°C) and the light side a temperature of +250°F (120°C)—giving the average temperature of 0°F—you likely would be quite upset with the travel agent for not giving you better information.[8] Likewise, the *average* surface

temperature of Earth may not mean much to you, as the actual temperature varies depending on where you're located. Even then, there's
still a lot of variability in any given location because of temperature
changes between day and night and summer and winter; there is also
temperature variability relative to passing storms. The point is, even
with all of this variability Earth's surface is consistently getting
warmer over time.

So, *how much* warmer? An increase between 2°F (1.1°C) and 11.5°F
(6.4°C) may not sound like much, but it is actually far more significant
than it appears. The average temperature of Earth's surface during the last
ice age, when glaciers a mile thick lay on top of what is now Manhattan,
was only 9°F (5°C) colder than it is now.[9] If a difference of only 9°F
colder made such an impact on our climate, we can count on even a few
degrees warmer to make a similarly huge difference. Because our climate
is temperature driven, and we're now moving into uncharted territory in
terms of how much $CO_2$ and other harmful levels of gases are in our
atmosphere, what that increase in average temperature really means is
that our climate is likely to become quite chaotic. As we said, those few
degrees of temperature rise will result in more extreme and destructive
weather events.[1]

## SEA LEVEL RISE

Then there's a potential rise in sea level of up to 2 feet (60 cm), which is
enough to flood many coastal areas, islands, and atolls. Although that
might not be absolutely devastating to most populated coastal areas, this
figure, unfortunately, takes into consideration only the melting of some of
the inland glaciers and the seas expanding because warm water takes up
more space than cold water.[1] While those are important considerations,
they do not take into account the very recent research that has uncovered how quickly Greenland's ice sheet and Antarctica are melting. If
both of these large bodies of ice melt completely, sea levels could rise
about 200 feet (70 meters).

Scientists don't think that *all* of Antarctica, which is twice the size of
Australia and is covered by an ice sheet about a mile thick, is likely to
melt any time soon. They are concerned, however, that Greenland's ice
sheet could melt quickly, which would cause the sea level to rise more
than 20 feet (3 meters). And parts of Antarctica, such as the West
Antarctic Ice Sheet, appear to be less stable than the rest. If the
West Antarctic Ice Sheet melts, that will raise sea levels another 20 or
more feet. We know from geologic records that when temperatures were

only 3.6°F to 5.4°F (2°C to 3°C) warmer than they are today, the sea
level was between 45 and 105 feet (14 to 32 meters) higher![10] That tells
us that if we continue to use fossil fuels and produce greenhouse gases
as we do now, causing temperatures to increase by as much as 11.5 °F
(6.4°C), we are condemning the world to losing *a lot* of coastline,
including the majority of the world's largest cities. We'll talk more
about sea level rise and what that means for our health in the chapter
on this topic.

Just so you know, part of the reason why Greenland and Antarctica are
melting faster than previously expected is because the Earth is warming
up more quickly at the poles than at the equator (there's that problem
with *averages* again!). Ocean currents carry warm, surface water to the
Arctic. While the *average* temperature of Earth has only warmed 1.4°F
(0.8°C) during the past century, the Arctic has warmed about 5°F
(2.8°C) during that time.[11]

## DANGEROUS CLIMATE CHANGE

You can tell from this information that global warming could get very
serious, and scientists have three criteria for "dangerous" climate change:

- Sea level rise of more than about three feet (1 meter)
- Greater than 50 percent extinction of species
- Regional climate change that severely compromises local food and water
  supplies

Dangerous climate change, according to the research, will very likely
occur with only 2°F (1.2°C) additional global warming above 2000 levels.
That amount of temperature increase corresponds to $CO_2$ levels of 450 ppm
in the atmosphere, and as of May 2008 the $CO_2$ level was 385 ppm. Global
greenhouse gas emissions increase every year. With current trends of
increasing emissions, we could reach that higher number by 2050. To prevent that, scientists say that our greenhouse gas emission levels must
decrease at least 20 percent by 2020 and 80 percent by 2050. Unfortunately, holding $CO_2$ levels at or below the 450 ppm level comes with no
guarantee that catastrophic climate chaos will be avoided. In fact, stabilizing $CO_2$ levels at 450 ppm gives us about a 50 percent chance of keeping
the global average temperature rise to a maximum of 3.6°F (2°C) above
preindustrial levels, or 2.6°F (1.4°C) above 2000 levels.[12] That means that
the goal of reducing $CO_2$ levels by 80 percent by 2050 should be seen as an
absolute minimum reduction.

To summarize all of this, the average temperature of our Earth's surface is increasing and, if left unchecked, it will likely be higher than it's been since humans first walked the land. Sea levels will increase at least one to two feet but likely much more than that in the next 50 to 100 years. And we can expect more extreme weather events. The bottom line is that we're looking at real climate chaos if we don't quickly and drastically change the way we now live.

## THE MOST WORRISOME GREENHOUSE GASES

Although we talk most about $CO_2$ because it makes up the largest proportion of the greenhouse gases emitted, not all greenhouse gases have the same capacity to hold the Sun's energy and cause global warming. Methane, which makes up only about 10 percent of all greenhouse gas emissions, is actually about 23 times more powerful than $CO_2$. The major source of methane is animal agriculture and decaying organic matter. Nitrogen oxides, which make up only 5 percent of the emissions, are almost 300 times more powerful.[12] Nitrogen oxides come primarily from vehicle tailpipes, but also from ships, trains, power plants, and some commercial and industrial processes.[13]

There are some other chemicals now in the atmosphere that we produced to replace what we thought were older atmosphere-harming chemicals. An example of one of the most damaging of these chemicals is called sulfur hexafluoride. It's used in electrical insulation and is more than 22,000 times as powerful as $CO_2$ at trapping the Sun's energy and heating up the Earth. Luckily, these chemicals only exist in very small quantities—only about 2 percent of all emissions—but they are so dangerous that they need to be carefully restricted to minimize their atmospheric damage.[12] Really, they should be phased out altogether as quickly as possible. This is an example of how solutions to one problem have caused more trouble elsewhere, namely for our climate. This demonstrates why we need to be vigilant about the unintended consequences of our efforts to solve problems of our own making. And climate change is one of our biggest problems ever.

## THE SPEED OF CLIMATE CHANGE

Although we've described climate change as gradual warming, there is strong geologic evidence that Earth's climate has had periods of very dramatic change. Climate scientists believe there are "thresholds" in the climate. Once a threshold is passed, changes happen very quickly and abruptly and are far more difficult to stop or alter. The National Academy of Sciences likens abrupt climate change to flipping a light switch.[14] This is an apt metaphor because if you break down the activity of flipping a light switch into a series of slow-motion events, you would see that you push and push and push on the switch, and initially nothing much happens. At this stage of the process, if you stop pushing the switch will return to its original position and the light stays off. If you continue to push, however, you will eventually cross a certain threshold in the light switch's path. Once past this threshold, the switch "flips" very rapidly to the other side and the light comes on. Once you cross the threshold, stopping the process of turning on the light becomes difficult, if not impossible, because the "flip" happens so quickly. Climate scientists believe similar thresholds exist in our climate. As the temperature warms past one of these thresholds, the climate could change rapidly and dramatically. The problem is we don't really know where these thresholds occur, but we do have some evidence and scientific theories about how the rapid changes might occur and what kinds of conditions might trigger these mechanisms. We will describe four of the most prominent mechanisms that climate scientists are especially concerned about:

- Melting ice—As the Sun's energy hits the surface of the Earth, some surfaces better reflect that energy back into space than others. You may know that light surfaces don't absorb as much heat as dark ones. Ice is very good at reflecting the Sun's energy, but as the ice melts from warming temperatures the dark surfaces of the sea and land under the ice get exposed and these absorb more heat. The more heat they absorb, the more the surface of the Earth warms and the more the ice melts, creating a positive feedback loop—except the outcome is anything but positive.
- More methane—In addition to absorbing more heat from the Sun, the other problem with the loss of Arctic ice is that the frozen remains of plants and animals can thaw. When that happens, the decomposition process halted by the freezing can resume, releasing large amounts of methane, which we've already learned is more potent than $CO_2$ as a greenhouse gas. The more methane released, the warmer the surface of the Earth gets, which releases more methane. Again, we have an unwelcome positive feedback loop.
- The ocean conveyor belt theory—As most of us live on land and only interact with the oceans when we go to the beach, we generally aren't aware that there are strong forces within the oceans at work moving vast quantities of water around—sometimes called the ocean conveyor belt. These water movements form strong currents of colder, saltier water in the depths

generally moving in one direction, and warmer, less salty water near the surface usually moving in a different direction. These currents influence the weather, forming, for example, the Trade Winds, which are important for ships plying the seas; these currents can also affect the climates of coastal areas. As the Arctic melts, large quantities of cold, fresh water are being dumped into the oceans, which could disrupt this ocean conveyor belt and change the climate quite abruptly in certain parts of the world. Western Europe, for example, could actually get *colder* than it is now. (This is one more reason why scientists prefer the term *climate change* to *global warming*.) Climate chaos, then, reflects the instability—not just warming—that will result with increased greenhouse gas emissions. Meanwhile, recent research shows that the Gulf Stream—the portion of the ocean conveyor belt in the Atlantic Ocean—is actually more variable than previously thought, too, and a new study deploying underwater sensors moored to the ocean floor will provide constant data that can alert the scientists if the current seems to be slowing.[15]

- *Loss of "carbon sinks"*—Plants absorb $CO_2$ as part of their photosynthesis process to capture the Sun's energy and turn it into chemical energy to grow. Plants in the oceans also absorb $CO_2$, and the ocean water itself absorbs some $CO_2$. These are called carbon sinks. As a result, the oceans and the land plants absorb about half of our $CO_2$ emissions. Unfortunately, the effects of climate change, along with the effects of human development, have degraded the ability of these carbon sinks to absorb $CO_2$. Without intervention, the degradation of carbon sinks is expected to worsen, meaning that more of our $CO_2$ emissions will go into the atmosphere to cause further warming and climate change, causing, in turn, more degradation to the carbon sinks, and so on.

## GREENHOUSE GAS EMISSIONS ACROSS NATIONS

Currently, the United States contributes about 20 percent of the global greenhouse gas emissions annually (6,868 million tons of $CO_2$ every year) but has about 4 percent of the global population. These emissions are divided by sector in Figure 2.3. Electricity production and heating is the largest category with 39 percent. Transportation is the next-largest category with 25 percent. These two categories, then, represent the largest possibilities for reductions in greenhouse gas emissions.

China is close behind the United States in total annual greenhouse gas emissions, with almost 14 percent of the global total (4,883 million tons of $CO_2$), and it is expected to be the major emitter in the very near future. This has provided some contention between the two countries during

# United States Greenhouse Gas Emissions by Sector for 2000

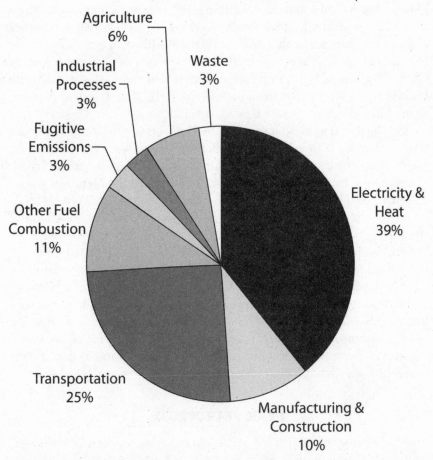

**Figure 2.3**   Source: Data for chart from Climate Analysis Indicators Tool, Version 5.0, World Resources Institute, Washington, DC.

negotiations of the Kyoto Protocol, a global treaty to reduce emissions. The U.S. negotiators have refused to ratify the treaty, saying that if China doesn't sign on to the Kyoto Protocol there's no point in the United States doing so because true global reductions won't occur. China, on the other hand, says it has a right to develop and acquire the same standard of living as the United States, and signing on to the Kyoto Protocol will keep it from achieving that goal. Both sides make good points, but we must consider additional information. The United States has been emitting greenhouse gases in substantial quantities for more than a century, while China has only been doing so for a relatively short time. That difference is reflected in cumulative emissions, which for the United States total about 28 percent of all greenhouse gas emissions since 1950 compared to China's cumulative emissions of 9 percent. Another important difference is that U.S. annual emissions per person are more than 24 tons of $CO_2$ versus slightly less than 4 tons of $CO_2$ per person in China. Yet China has a population that is four times greater than the United States, so if it uses fossil fuels to reach the same standard of living as the United States climate chaos is assured.[16]

The biggest reason that neither of their arguments hold up under serious scrutiny is that if drastic reductions in greenhouse gas emissions aren't made right away, everyone on the planet will suffer from climate chaos. These two countries are acting like intoxicated teenagers racing their cars head on toward each other in a game of "chicken." Honor might dictate that neither one be the first to swerve, but that kind of thinking gets everyone killed.

Because the United States has contributed the most to global warming, it is logical for it to be the first to "swerve" and avert total destruction for all. The United States and other industrial countries have the financial and technical resources to help China and other developing countries improve their standards of living without following the same destructive fossil fuel-burning pathways they did. Moreover, U.S. citizens and institutions have a solemn responsibility to do everything in their power to stabilize the climate and prevent climate chaos.

## PEAK PETROLEUM

We have another major obstacle to reducing our greenhouse gas emissions. Petroleum is a finite resource and many respected scientists, including petroleum geologists and energy industry analysts, project that we will reach the peak of petroleum production soon, if we have not already done so. Although there is some uncertainty, and thus debate, about when this will occur, there is no argument that it will occur eventually. The majority of analysts predict the year of peak production will be between 2005 and 2010, but a clear signal of peak production cannot be discerned until a few years after it has been passed. Despite increasing global demand, oil production has remained steady for the past several years.

Once we have passed the peak, termed *after peak oil* or *peak petroleum* by various analysts, petroleum production is predicted to decline 3–5 percent annually. Thus there will be a growing mismatch between increasing demand and falling production, so petroleum prices will rise dramatically. This increased cost will be manifest in many ways. It will include higher prices for a barrel of crude oil and higher prices for gasoline as well as for consumer products dependent on petroleum, such as everything containing plastic. Higher food prices are expected, too, because our current agricultural industry relies on petroleum to run the farm machinery, produce the fertilizers and pesticides used on crops, and transport the food to central processing plants and markets. Construction costs are also expected to rise because construction materials require large amounts of petroleum to manufacture and transport.

Although at first glance the idea of running out of the very fossil fuel that has caused much of our climate-change woes might seem like a timely "fix" for this situation, the reality is that as the price of crude oil increases, the possibility of extracting oil from nontraditional sources, including oil sands and oil shale, becomes more economically appealing. These nontraditional sources require far more energy to extract, resulting in even greater greenhouse gas emissions per unit of energy derived and higher environmental and health costs. Moreover, because coal still exists in large supply, using more relatively inexpensive coal with its higher greenhouse gas emissions will certainly doom us to climate chaos.

Land use, food production and distribution, water use, transportation networks, transportation patterns, building design, product design, and the notion of globalization itself have all been developed with readily available, inexpensive, petroleum-based energy. Because our society has been fully constructed to depend on an endless supply of inexpensive oil, the eventual lack of it will have profound effects on all aspects of our society.

Moreover, projections of greenhouse gas emissions over time have generally not factored in the increased emissions from the use of more coal or of nontraditional fossil fuels as the demand for energy outstrips the supply of oil. The complex set of solutions that must be implemented to slow climate change have not, to date, factored in the economic, political, social, and environmental constraints and pressures that will result from this new era of increasingly expensive energy.

Any hope of successfully achieving needed greenhouse gas emission reduction goals, then, will depend on effectively avoiding the "easy" energy shortage solutions of relying on more coal or encouraging the use of nontraditional fossil fuels. Peak petroleum clearly presents a huge challenge in its own right and must be considered along with the challenge of avoiding climate chaos so that solutions to one problem don't worsen the other.

Although there are some actions you can take to reduce risk of illness or injury from climate change—and these will be covered in the subsequent chapters—no amount of adapting will prevent the extensive, catastrophic changes that will take place if the climate is not stabilized. If emissions are not curtailed, global warming will cause the climate to become so chaotic that completely protecting yourself or your family will be impossible.

## THE BOOK'S OUTLINE

Now that you have a basic understanding of how climate change occurs, let's take a quick look at what you will learn in the ensuing chapters about how climate change could harm your health. Each chapter ends with a solutions section that can help you protect yourself and prevent climate chaos.

## Chapter 3: Temperature: Home Is Getting Hotter

More frequent heat waves that will last longer and attain higher temperatures will be one of the hallmarks of climate change. Some people are more vulnerable to heat than others, including babies, children, the elderly, the poor, and those who live in inner-city neighborhoods. Prior to Hurricane Katrina, more people died from heat stress than from any other weather-related event in the United States. With more frequent and severe heat waves, we can expect more deaths and heat-related illnesses, especially in these vulnerable groups. In this chapter, we'll talk about what happens to our bodies when they overheat and the various stages of heat stress, including what to watch out for and do if someone gets overheated. We'll also look at how heat affects behavior.

## Chapter 4: Air: Breathing Harder

As temperatures rise, ozone—the primary component of what we call smog—gets worse. Ozone is bad for our health because it damages our lungs and hearts. People who have asthma suffer the most from ozone, having a harder time breathing and requiring more medicine to keep their breathing controlled. Sometimes they end up in an emergency room or hospital if the medicines can't keep up with the damage the ozone is doing. People who don't have asthma suffer from ozone as well. Other kinds of air pollution will also get worse with climate change and play an important role in heart and lung disease. In this chapter, we'll discuss the ways that climate change will affect air quality and how that can harm our health. We'll also address how air pollution may influence how we behave.

## Chapter 5: Water: Water, Water
### Everywhere or Neverthere

As the average temperature of Earth's surface increases with global warming, precipitation patterns will change. Some regions will get wetter, but many will get drier overall. Erratic weather will be more common, too, and may cause more rain and flooding one year and then extreme drought for several years thereafter. Water certainly is vital to life, and apart from having enough clean water to drink we use it for a variety of tasks important to our health. Without sufficient clean water to grow our food, keep our bodies clean, and cook and wash the dishes, it is harder to stay healthy. In this chapter, we'll explore the many ways that climate change will affect the quality and quantity of our water supply and the ways those changes will affect our health. We'll also address how failing to have enough clean water can affect our mental well-being.

## Chapter 6: Cataclysmic Events: Pounding
### People and the Planet

Climate change will cause sea levels to rise as a result of the expansion of the seas from increased temperature, melting of inland glaciers, and the melting of the polar ice caps. As sea levels rise, coastal areas will be at increased risk for inundation as well as flooding from storm surge during extreme weather events, such as hurricanes. Flooding causes a variety of ill effects to our health, including death by drowning, injuries, problems from mold, toxins in the water, and saltwater contamination of freshwater wells, to name a few. In this chapter, we'll cover a range of health consequences of sea level rise, hurricanes, flooding, and other cataclysmic weather events, including how being displaced from our homes and ancestral lands by these events may affect our long-term mental health.

## Chapter 7: Infectious Disease: Bacteria,
### Viruses, and Parasites, Oh My

Many infectious diseases are known to increase or decrease with climate trends. Insect-borne diseases are especially sensitive to changes in temperature, humidity, and rainfall patterns. In this chapter, we'll summarize the current research on which diseases are expected to become more of a problem in different regions of the United States and around the world and what individuals can do to reduce their risk of catching one of these diseases. We'll also address how climate-related infectious diseases can harm our mental health.

## Chapter 8: Food: Nature's Bounty Bashed

Plants require certain amounts of moisture and nutrients and can only live in particular temperature ranges. A warmer climate and changes in precipitation patterns, then, will no doubt have major effects on the global food supply. In this chapter, we will explore how the ranges of specific food crops may change. We'll also discuss how oil will become more scarce and expensive, which, in concert with climate change, will further harm our food supplies if we don't make substantive changes to how we manage our food in the future. Proper nourishment, certainly, is important to how we behave, too, and we'll touch on this as well.

## Chapter 9: Ecosystem Health: Cycles of Life . . . Or Death

An ecosystem is a community of different species of plants and animals interdependent on each other and their environment, and each ecosystem is distinct from neighboring communities of plants and animals. Different types of ecosystems are often defined by the dominant species found within them—for example, forest ecosystems, prairie ecosystems, or coral reef ecosystems. Each of these ecosystems provides "services" to humans, such as clean air, clean water, and food. In spite of all the modern technology we've created, we are still reliant on these ecosystems to provide the basic necessities of life. Many of Earth's ecosystems are already stressed by human activities, such as pollution or suburban encroachment. Climate change will be another huge stress and has the potential to provide the last straw for some ecosystems. We'll look at how the health of Earth's ecosystems is important to our own health, what could happen if ecosystems were to collapse because of climate change's impacts, and how our health could be severely compromised as a result. We'll explore how our energy choices affect the well-being of ecosystems and suggest some of the things we can do to prevent ecosystem collapse.

## Chapter 10: Human Behavior: Choice to Change

While we have known about climate change and its potential for devastating harm to us and our planet for years, we have done almost nothing to prevent that harm. Certainly people are concerned about climate change and express a desire to deter it—and we have some tools at our disposal to do so—but our patterns of consumption have actually increased $CO_2$ emissions in recent years more than ever before. This chapter will explore some of the individual and community factors that have allowed us to avoid changing our behavior to curb global warming and how we might be able to make new choices that actually begin to prevent our climate-damaging behavior.

## Chapter 11: Epilogue

Despite everything you may have read, seen, or heard about climate change and the risks it holds in store for the health of humanity and the planet, we do have another way. This chapter will present an alternative tale of hope for us to change the ways we live to avert climate chaos.

# Chapter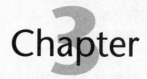

## Temperature:
## Home Is Getting Hotter

Maria is sweating. She had hours ago given up the struggle to get the cluttered, tiny den ready for her two nieces and two nephews and went to the kitchen to make dinner, but even without much exertion now she notices drops of moisture falling from her brow, and her shirt is damp. She checks the temperature in the house. The thermostat reads 80°F (26.7°C). Maria has kept it there because of the local restrictions on overuse of air conditioning, even though she could safely turn it down a few more degrees. Then she looks at the outdoor temperature on a digital thermometer device Moravia bought recently: 114°F (45.6°C). Maria shakes her head. "It's 7 pm and still so hot," she says softly to herself. "No wonder so many of my patients are sick."

When she opens the refrigerator to collect the vegetables Moravia earlier cut into small pieces for the pasta sauce she plans to make, she lingers for a moment in the blast of cool air. Then she turns on the radio to hear the news. "More than 160 people in the region, mostly the elderly and some children, have died from heat-related illness in the past three days," the radio announcer intones, "and two of the six day-time cooling shelters have had to close down because they have run out of money to stay open. City leaders are asking citizens to remain calm and stay out of the heat as best they can and again are recommending that you drink plenty of fluids, watch. . . ."

Maria stares at the radio, listening to the list of common precautions that follow. The pattern of astronomic heat and death has persisted for weeks, and nothing seems to be truly helping. And she thinks, this is what Max wants to live with now? This is the way it's going to be for us? She shakes her head slowly and turns on a burner to make the sauce.

## IT COULD GET HOT

More than 140 Californians succumbed to a blistering heat wave in July 2006, and some health officials raised concerns that the toll was as much as three times higher. The same heat wave took 140 lives in New York City and in other cities across the nation. Meanwhile, August 2007 saw more heat waves across the United States, with 44 deaths reported in the South.

During two days in late July 2007, scorching heat killed five people in Greece while four people died in Romania during a heat wave that gripped Southeast Europe. Tourists died on the beaches in Turkey where temperatures reached 111° F (44°C). Brush fires broke out in southern Italy and all over Greece, where temperatures topped 104°F (40°C).

Maybe you think a few deaths and fires from deadly heat waves aren't a big deal. So consider that in 2003 in Western Europe a massive heat wave killed 45,000 people in just a few days. If climate chaos occurs unabated, by 2040 heat waves as severe as that one could occur every other year.[1]

Clearly, we already are seeing the early effects of global warming on temperatures across the United States and around the world. Seven of the eight warmest years on record have occurred since 2001, and the 10 warmest years have occurred since 1997.[2] Computer models tell us that average global surface temperatures will get hotter during the coming decades. That means that there will be fewer cold days, spring will generally come earlier in the year, summer will last longer, and fall will end later in the year.

Heat waves, defined as three or more consecutive days with temperatures at least 90°F (32.2°C), will become more frequent, intense, and longer lasting than ever before.[3,4] Overall, heat waves are expected to occur with the greatest intensity in the Southeast and Western United States, as well as Western Europe and the Mediterranean.[4] Still, average summer temperatures in the eastern United States may increase by nearly 10°F (5.6°C) by the 2080s, and summers that have lower than average rainfall would likely be the hottest. Cities such as Washington, DC, Atlanta, and even Chicago could see daily high temperatures between 100°F (37.8°C) and 110°F (43.3°C) during the driest summers.[5]

Many of these predictions come from commonly used computer model projections of expected temperatures in North America and across the globe that use the "heat index," which is a combination of the temperature and the humidity. The heat index more accurately reflects what a human body feels because when the humidity is high, it feels hotter at a given temperature than when there is little humidity.

So, what do we do when the heat gets to be so scorching in the United States, Europe, and other places on the planet? We turn up our air conditioners! That's what happened in Southeast Europe during the summer heat wave of 2007, and it caused massive blackouts. Although air conditioning may keep the heat from harming us at the moment, the electricity it uses makes climate change worse because most of our electricity is generated from fossil fuels that spew $CO_2$ into the atmosphere. We'll continue to need air conditioning—even more so than we do now—making it that much more important that our electricity be generated from clean, renewable sources that don't contribute to the climate change problem. We'll also need to markedly improve the efficiency of air conditioners, and we'll likely need to get used to not having our living spaces over-air conditioned so that using them doesn't cause deadly blackouts.

## HEAT AND OUR HEALTH

Frequent heat waves already kill a lot of people around the world. One of the deadliest heat waves in the United States occurred in 1995 when Chicago experienced a 4-day span of high temperatures and humidity that killed more than 700 people.[6]

The summer 2003 heat wave in Western Europe was the most deadly in recorded history.[7] It's difficult to comprehend how 45,000 people could die from heat stress in developed countries when air conditioning is prevalent and modern medical care is available, isn't it? The worst part of that summer's heat wave began on August 4 when temperatures hit 99°F (37°C) in a region of the world where temperatures are usually much more temperate. The heat wave continued nine straight days until August 13. Researchers have determined that during the past 125 years, Western Europe has had three times as many hot days, and the length of summer heat waves has doubled.[8]

The length of time temperatures stay high is important for how much the human body is able to adapt to the heat because the effects of heat are cumulative. During heat waves, nighttime temperatures also stay high, preventing the body from cooling down and recuperating.

Nighttime temperatures in Ohio, for example, have consistently climbed during the past 50 years, partly due to higher humidity levels.[9] Most people can take a day or two of high temperatures, but when a heat wave continues three or more days, the most vulnerable people start to succumb. More about this in a moment. Heat waves also make certain kinds of air pollution, such as ground-level ozone, worse, and this appears to play an important role in why so many people die during heat waves.[10]

The human body is quite adept at maintaining a constant body temperature right around 98.6°F (37°C). To warm up, it narrows blood vessels to limit heat leaving from the skin, and it starts shivering to generate heat. To cool down, blood vessels near the skin get wider to let heat out, and the skin starts sweating. When all goes well, we're barely aware of this process. The body's ability to regulate temperature, however, can be overwhelmed by a hot external environment. The external heat itself, or coupled with exercise or heavy work that generates internal body heat, can result in *heat stress*.

Heat stress starts as mild overheating. Athletes and those doing heavy work in a hot environment can suffer from *heat cramps* caused by the blood vessels widening to dissipate the excess heat. The cramps are actually muscle spasms, and even though they can occur in any muscles they usually occur in the muscles of the arms, legs, and abdomen. They typically go away as soon as a person stops the vigorous exercise, cools down, and replaces lost fluids. If this doesn't happen, the heat cramps can progress to *heat exhaustion*, but not everyone who gets heat exhaustion gets heat cramps first.

People experiencing heat exhaustion may feel dizzy, weak, or very tired. Heat exhaustion can also cause nausea and vomiting, heavy sweating, quick and shallow breathing, and a fast and weak pulse. Sometimes the skin of a person suffering from heat exhaustion might even feel cool and moist, but that doesn't mean they're not overheated on the inside! Treatment of heat exhaustion may require hospitalization, and must include replacing fluids and salts and gently cooling the body.[3]

*Heat stroke*, which requires an internal body temperature of at least 105°F (40.6°C), is the most serious and life-threatening form of heat stress, and it qualifies as a medical emergency. Heat stroke is characterized by feeling too weak or lethargic to move, being disoriented, and suffering pounding headaches. The skin will usually feel hot and dry. Heat stroke can also come on abruptly; victims may not experience any of these heralding symptoms.[11] Without emergency medical attention, heat stroke can rapidly progress to delirium and eventually a coma. Even if heat stroke victims are taken to a hospital and rapidly cooled, damage to their brains and nervous systems can be severe and irreparable.[3] Following the Chicago heat wave in 1995, about a third of those who experienced heat stroke had severe brain injuries and died within a year as a result.[12]

## THE MOST VULNERABLE TO HEAT STRESS

Infants, children, and the elderly are especially vulnerable to heat stress. Infants are more vulnerable because they have more skin surface area compared to their body mass, and that allows them to heat up more quickly. Another problem for infants in a hot environment is that they can't move themselves to a cooler place. They must rely on adults to notice that they are getting over-heated and take care of the problem.

Children are more vulnerable to heat stress than adults because they often don't notice that they are becoming overheated. They run and play, producing more internal heat, even when temperatures are high, and that causes them to heat up more quickly. In addition, they often play outside where the temperatures may be hottest, and they are less able to dissipate heat because they don't sweat as much as adults.[11]

It is the elderly, however, who are at the greatest risk of heat stress for a variety of reasons. Medically, the elderly are more apt to suffer from heart conditions that limit their bodies' ability to compensate for overheating. When the body's internal temperature gets too high and the blood vessels near the surface of the skin widen to allow the heat to dissipate, the heart needs to beat more quickly and strongly to maintain adequate blood pressure. If the heart is not strong and healthy, it can have trouble keeping up with the demand. This not only results in reduced heat dissipation, but could also result in dizziness, passing out, or a heart attack.

The elderly also are more likely to be taking medications that blunt their bodies' responses to overheating, such as sweating and feeling thirsty to encourage drinking more fluids. An elderly person can progress from heat exhaustion to heat stroke in just a few minutes without intervention. Social conditions can also put the elderly at higher risk. They are more likely to be socially isolated with no one to make sure they drink extra fluids or turn on air conditioning, and problems with mobility can prevent elderly people from physically moving to a cooler environment, such as an air-conditioned shopping mall or shelter. In France, researchers found that people who were more dependent on others to accomplish their daily routines were more apt to have died during the heat wave in 2003. This was particularly true for people living in the community as opposed to a facility like a nursing home.[13]

During the Chicago heat wave of 1995, people older than 65 were 14 times more likely to die than their younger counterparts.[14] During Europe's heat wave in 2003, 82 percent of the victims in France who succumbed to heat stress were more than 75 years old.[13] Age alone, however, doesn't compromise people's ability to tolerate or acclimate to the heat if they exercise well and don't have other illnesses.[15]

The fourth group of people who are more vulnerable to heat stress consists of people of any age who suffer from any kind of pre-existing medical conditions, such as heart and lung diseases, cancer, mental illness, diseases of the nervous system, or diseases of the immune system, particularly if the diseases confine them to their beds, as was found during the 1995 heat wave in Chicago.[6] The numbers of people dying as a result of heat waves may be underestimated because death rates for other diseases also increase during heat waves.[16] Other risk factors include living on a building's top floor, having no air conditioning (fans don't protect people from dying), having no transportation, and especially experiencing social isolation. Social isolation is such a strong risk factor that during the Chicago heat wave, researchers found that the risk of death was decreased by almost anything that aided social contact, even membership in a social club or owning a pet.[6]

Even healthy people who don't fall into any of the aforementioned four groups can still get heat stress and even heat stroke. Heavy exertion in a hot environment can cause heat stress that can then progress to heat stroke if the body does not get a chance to cool. Studies show that the higher the temperature and the harder the work, the less work time is possible before workers collapse from the heat.[17]

Athletes, perhaps the healthiest people, must also be careful not to exercise too much in extreme heat. This was demonstrated in the fall of 2007 when more than 300 Chicago marathon runners needed ambulances to pick them up and treat them for heat stress, many requiring hospitalization. For the first time in the history of the Chicago Marathon, officials called off the race before noon when temperatures topped 88°F (31°C).

## POVERTY: ANOTHER RISK FACTOR FOR HEAT STRESS

The most immediate solution for surviving a heat wave is to spend as much time as possible in an air-conditioned space. People living in poverty may not have the financial resources to buy an air conditioner, or they may be concerned that they will not be able to pay the added electricity costs. Some who died during the Chicago heat wave had air conditioners but refused to use them for fear their electricity would be shut off if they couldn't pay the added cost to run the air conditioners. Poor people often also don't have transportation to get to a shelter or an air-conditioned facility, such as a shopping mall. Unfortunately, the two most vulnerable groups, the elderly and children, are disproportionately represented in the nation's poor, compounding an already severe problem. Thirty-nine percent of all children live in low-income families and 10 percent of people older than 65 live in poverty.[18,19]

## GEOGRAPHY MATTERS

People living in cities experience hotter temperatures because of something called the *urban heat island effect*. Cities are created from massive amounts of cement and asphalt with many dark surfaces that absorb the heat from the sun all day. This makes them hotter during the day, and then all that hot mass of cement and asphalt radiates heat throughout the night, keeping nighttime temperatures high. Even though trees and plants can keep surrounding areas much cooler, many cities aren't known for having huge numbers of trees and plants, compounding the urban heat island effect. As you can see in Figure 3.1, rural areas tend to be the coolest, then suburban areas, with urban areas being the warmest. Researchers have found that temperatures can be up to 20°F (11°C) warmer in some major cities compared to surrounding rural areas.[20]

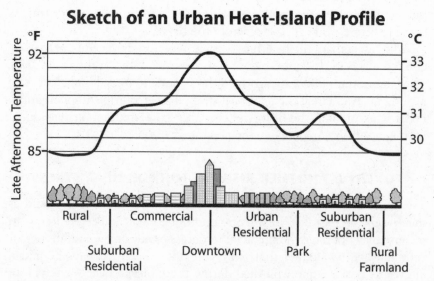

**Figure 3.1**   Source: Graphic produced and used with permission by Heat Island Group at the Lawrence Berkeley National Laboratory.

Where on the map you are also makes a difference. Heat waves generally hit northern cities harder than southern cities. During the Chicago heat wave, for example, the temperatures were not much different from what they typically are during a Phoenix summer, but far more people died in Chicago than typically die from the heat every summer in Phoenix. This is probably because people living in southern areas are already used to the heat. Their bodies may have adapted some, but most of the adaptation has likely been in their behaviors. More southern homes and buildings have air conditioning, and people have already figured out what to do when the temperatures soar. In central and northern cities, on the other hand, many people do not have air conditioning in their homes because, up until recently, they rarely needed it, and most people do not have a conscious plan to deal with potential heat waves. Northern cities suffered more than southern cities in Italy, England, and Wales during the 2003 heat wave in Western Europe.[21,22]

Examining all heat-related deaths in the United States, researchers found that cities in the north-central states suffered greater mortality from heat waves, followed by those in the northeast. The southern states and those along the Pacific coast were the least affected. Cities that are not located on a coast are also at greater risk because the oceans tend to help moderate the temperatures, keeping coastal communities from getting as hot.[23] Figures 3.2 and 3.3 give us some idea of what is expected by 2100 in different areas of the United States if global warming is allowed to continue.

## GENDER CONSIDERATIONS

During the 1995 Chicago heat wave, elderly men were two and a half times more likely to die than elderly women.[24] Other heat waves, however, have shown that women are slightly more likely to die during a heat wave than men.[22]

Sweating helps cool the body through evaporation, but only if the humidity is low. Women tend to have higher "sweat thresholds," meaning they don't start sweating until the temperature gets hotter than the level it typically takes for men to start sweating. This gives women a slight advantage in a hot, humid environment because they're not wasting precious body fluids producing sweat that won't help them cool off. Conversely, men have a slight advantage in hot, dry environments because they sweat more, and the evaporation of the sweat cools them off. These minor differences, however, are measurable in a laboratory setting but probably aren't noticeable in a real-world setting. Even the hormonal changes associated with the menstrual cycle don't noticeably alter an otherwise physically fit woman's ability to perform work in the heat. Overall work performance in hot

## Projected Dec-Jan-Feb Temperature Changes
## for 2091-2100

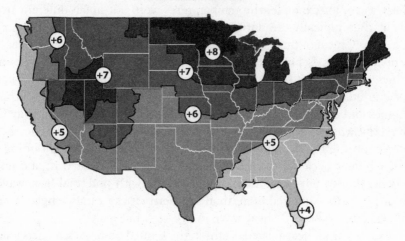

Figure 3.2

## Projected Jun-Jul-Aug Temperature Changes
## for 2091-2100

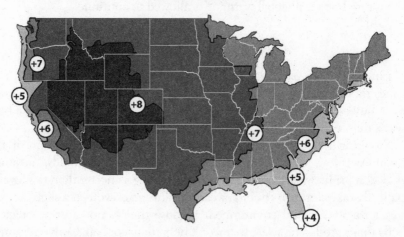

**Figure 3.3** These maps show the changes in temperature increases in degrees Fahrenheit relative to 1971–2000 averages for the United States if we do not reduce greenhouse gas emissions. Figure 3.2 shows projected wintertime temperature increases and Figure 3.3 shows projected summertime temperature increases. Source: JL Weiss, The University of Arizona, with data from Hoerling & Eischeid NOAA ESRL.

temperatures has far more to do with how fit a person is than his or her gender. Research shows that those who are more physically fit, lean, and participate in regular cardiovascular exercise are better able to handle the heat.[15] This is another good reason to exercise regularly!

It is possible to adapt—or acclimate—to hot environments, however. Athletes exercising in the heat and workers performing heavy labor in the heat at least three to four days per week do gradually improve their heat tolerance.[15]

## RACE AND ETHNICITY

During the 1995 Chicago heat wave, Hispanics, who made up 23 percent of the population at that time, contributed only 2 percent of the heat-related deaths. The reason for this is unclear.[24] African Americans, on the other hand, were 50 percent more likely to die from the heat than their white counterparts. This situation was thought to be the result, more likely, of poverty than of any actual difference in how people's bodies handle the heat. Because various ethnic groups originated in different climates, it would seem reasonable to suspect genetic differences in how different groups handle the heat. That, however, doesn't seem to be the case. Apparently, all humans essentially function like tropical animals. Significant individual differences in heat and cold tolerance do occur, but these differences don't extend to an entire ethnic group.

## FEWER DEATHS FROM COLD WEATHER?

Okay, so maybe you're thinking that if the climate gets warmer, it's reasonable to expect fewer deaths from extreme cold. In general, that's true, although global climate change is more than just a steady, gentle warming. Because our climate is temperature driven, it is changing and becoming less stable. Some areas of the globe could actually get colder. Overall, however, most areas will get warmer and fewer people will die from extreme cold events. Many who die during the winter, however, don't die from exposure to extreme cold but from winter diseases such as influenza. New research suggests that lower temperatures and lower humidity facilitate the transmission of the influenza virus, at least among guinea pigs in a laboratory.[25] Further research is needed to know if a shorter winter season and warmer winter temperatures will reduce the thousands of deaths that occur every year from this disease. The increase in winter humidity might negate the effect. Unfortunately, the number of people projected to succumb to heat stress is far greater than those projected to be saved by milder winters.

## GLOBAL WARMING AND BEHAVIOR

In addition to the dangers to your health that a warming planet portends, it may worsen your behavior and mental health. First, there is little research on how heat waves affect our mental functioning, but it appears that heat waves may contribute to more alcohol and other substance abuse, more visits to emergency rooms for mental health problems, and even the possibility of being more dangerous toward others.[26,27]

Research has found associations between higher temperatures and an increased risk for more aggressive and violent behaviors, including behaviors categorized as assaults, rapes, robberies, and burglaries.[28–31] Just an increase of 1°F (0.5°C) shows evidence of significantly more criminal misbehavior.[29]

The reasons for the temperature-violence link are varied. Some speculate that warmer temperatures may actually affect people's brains through changes in stress hormones that lead to violent behavior.[31] Heat may also engender more irritability and hostility and lead to aggressive thoughts and behavior.[32,33] Another likely reason for the association between higher temperatures and more aggression and violence is that as it becomes warmer outside, people are more likely to leave their homes and spend time outdoors in their communities. By simply having more people interacting as a result of this temperature change, the risk for interpersonal aggression and other forms of violence may increase.[29] Of course, truly brutal heat might keep many people indoors . . . if they have access to air conditioning. In poorer communities, extreme heat may drive many people out of their overheated homes.

You might benefit from knowing that increased contact with nature, such as visits to nearby parks, appears to lessen human aggression by reducing the mental fatigue of living in stressful places.[34,35] Increased contact with nature in our communities could therefore reduce some of climate change's heat-induced violence. But for the many millions of people who live in inner-city areas devoid of accessible natural landscapes—and who also tend to experience more noise, crowding, limited resources, and other problems that can fuel violence—this benefit may be sorely lacking. In this light, it would seem prudent to work hard to prevent climate change's risks for our increased violent behavior.

## SOLUTIONS

### Individual

To protect yourself from heat stress during extreme heat:

- Drink plenty of cool liquids. Iced drinks are not as useful because they slow down drinking. And don't wait until you're feeling thirsty; keep drinking throughout the day. Avoid alcoholic as well as caffeinated beverages, such as coffee, tea, and soft drinks, because they can actually cause you to urinate more than you're drinking, resulting in dehydration. Sports drinks or salt pills are generally not required or useful for non-athletes and can be harmful.
- Check with your doctor before heat waves if you take "water pills" or are on restricted fluid intake for medical reasons. If you are an athlete or regularly engage in heavy work in a hot environment, also check with your doctor about what kind of fluids to drink and the best timing for fluid replacement.
- Stay indoors in air-conditioned rooms if possible, especially during the hottest part of the day. If you don't have air conditioning in your home, go to an air-conditioned facility, such as a shopping mall or a public library. Even a few hours a day in an air-conditioned place can be protective.
- If you are unable to be in an air-conditioned space, avoid strenuous activity. Rest is best.
- Wear lightweight, light-colored, loose clothing, and a wide-brimmed hat if you must go outside, and stay in the shade as much as possible.
- Use an electric fan, but remember that you can still get over-heated with just a fan.
- Take frequent cool showers, baths, or sponge-baths.
- Pregnant women should consult with their doctors before engaging in heavy activity in a hot environment.
- Plant trees around where you live to shade buildings.
- Put a white roof on your home to keep your house cooler.

If you have friends, relatives, or neighbors in one of the vulnerable groups discussed in this chapter, you can help them protect themselves by:

- Checking on them at least twice a day to make sure they are keeping cool.
- Providing a plentiful supply of cool liquids within easy reach.
- Helping them get to an air-conditioned place if necessary.

- Checking their body temperature with a thermometer. Normal body temperature is 98.6°F (37°C). If their temperature is above 99°F (37.2°C), it could mean that they aren't handling the heat well. Make arrangements to move them to a cooler place.
- If you find someone who may be suffering from heat stroke, call 911 immediately. While waiting for emergency professionals to arrive, move the person to a safe, cool, and well-ventilated place; remove unnecessary clothing; pour some cool water onto the skin and clothing; and fan vigorously. Some experts believe that cooling the face and head may promote brain cooling and prevent brain damage.[11]

## Community

- Many cities in the United States and in Europe have developed heat stress response plans. These involve local weather services that notify the health department to expect a heat wave. The health department then activates its heat stress plan, which typically involves, at a minimum, setting up cooling shelters.
- Some cities also notify home health services, such as home nursing agencies and Meals-on-Wheels, to check on their clients' ability to safely stay at home during heat waves or to help facilitate their removal to a cooling center, given that vulnerable people often have problems that prevent them from getting to cooler environments or shelters.
- You can get involved in these efforts by becoming part of a neighborhood, religious, or social group that checks on and helps vulnerable citizens, especially the elderly and children who don't realize they are becoming dangerously overheated. Know of places, even your own home, to take them to cool off to prevent heat stroke.[36]
- You may want to see if your utility companies will suspend all shut-offs during heat waves and suspend or reduce charges for electricity during heat waves to low-income residents to prevent tragic deaths that occur when some indigent people are afraid to use their air conditioners because of the added cost.
- Other actions a community can take include changing building codes to require every hotel, apartment building, nursing home, and assisted-living facility to have an air-conditioned lobby or common area. As access to air conditioning for only a few hours a day has been shown to be protective, this relatively simple act could save countless lives.[36]

Consider Philadelphia, which has a great heat stress plan. When the weather service notifies the city of a potential heat wave, the city puts relevant information on the radio and television stations; the health department contacts nursing homes and other entities that provide housing to high-risk individuals; local utilities halt service suspensions; fire and ambulance services increase staffing; senior centers extend their hours to serve as cooling centers; and homeless services extend their outreach. Independent reviewers determined that Philadelphia's heat warning system is highly cost effective. Between 1995 and 1998, an estimated 117 lives were saved: the benefits in lives saved far outweigh the costs.[37]

In a review of 18 U.S. cities that are especially at risk for heat-related deaths, one-third had no heat planning whatsoever, and most of those that did have plans were deemed to have major problems.[38] Ask your health department what their plan is to protect people during a heat wave. Make sure it includes all the points we've been talking about as well as adequate measures to get newspapers, radio, and especially television stations to broadcast messages of advice and instructions for how to take care of yourself and others during a heat wave.

## Reducing Your Community's Urban Heat Island Effect

Urban areas don't *have* to have higher temperatures:

- By planting more greenery throughout the city, increasing parks and other open green spaces, and reducing dark-colored surfaces, temperatures in urban areas can be closer to suburban or rural areas.
- Painting black-tar roofs with special white (best for keeping temperatures down) or silver (less expensive and still helps to reduce temperatures somewhat) roofing materials helps reduce city temperatures *and cools the insides of the buildings themselves*. These materials are available in home-improvement stores, allowing individual homeowners to change the color of their own roofs and save energy and money in cooling costs.
- Communities can take advantage of federal, and sometimes state and local, funding programs that provide money to low-income families to make their homes more energy efficient by, for example, installing white roofs.

Real estate is at a premium in cities, but buildings can provide acres of plantable surfaces—on their roofs! Chicago is leading the way in greening the city and installing these "green" roofs. Once a flat roof has been modified to hold the additional weight, soil can be placed on the roof and a variety of plants planted. Green roofs can even be used to grow food. Chicago has more than 250 green roofs planned or constructed, including City Hall.[39] In addition to reducing the urban heat island effect, green roofs reduce run-off of storm water, reduce the energy needed to air condition a building, and provide plants to absorb more $CO_2$, thereby further reducing global climate change.

## Regional, National, International

Even if we stop $CO_2$ emissions immediately, temperatures will still get at least another degree warmer. Air conditioning will be needed. The only way to use life-saving air conditioning without making the climate change problem worse is to switch to clean, renewable energy sources and to make air conditioners as efficient as possible. Help elect policy makers who will work to ensure our electricity is generated from clean, renewable sources and our appliances are energy efficient.

# Chapter 4

## Air: Breathing Harder

It's been bad enough that Zach's asthma has been acting up so severely this summer that Maria and Moravia are endlessly on edge and ready to dash him to the emergency room to prevent that one nightmarish, life-threatening attack that has yet to materialize. Maria also has been uneasy about Keisha, whose breathing problems aren't so bad but who seems more irritable and withdrawn, especially when the heat blazes higher and higher and the air seems thick and oppressive. Then, as Maria is putting together the pasta for dinner, she receives a call from her good friend Penny.

"Did you hear about the Ambley Flats Coal Plant?" Penny says, a little shriller than usual. Maria is uneasy again.

"No, no, I didn't, Pen. Sounds like it isn't good. . . ."

"Isn't good at all," Penny continues. "The EPA just found out—it was on the 6 pm news—that Ambley's been lying about how much junk is coming out of its smokestacks. That's just a few miles west of here!"

"You're kidding," Maria hears herself saying, although she knows there's no joke. She instinctively looks up to about where Zach's bedroom is on the floor above her.

"No, no, no," Penny replies. "Tons of soot, carbon dioxide, and other stuff. Much more than they've put down in their paperwork for the past couple years. They're saying that's one of the reasons so many people are having trouble breathing around here. Can you believe it?"

Maria doesn't answer. She's thinking mostly of Zach and of her brother and his family coming to live with them in just a few days. She's wondering how they're all going to make it with this rotten climate change and now the foul air they've been breathing.

"There's a link," Maria hears Penny saying.

"A what?" Maria replies.

"A link. The coal and the air and the heat and our breathing . . . "

"Yeah," Maria says flatly, staring out the kitchen window at the barren yard. "A link."

## THE CLIMATE–AIR POLLUTION CONNECTION

Climate change will worsen air quality. That's because air quality is the result of such effects as local wind speed and direction, precipitation, humidity, and barometric pressure, and climate change is expected to change all of those factors.

That's not to say we have no control over the situation. Air quality also depends a lot on what chemicals, toxins, and fine particulates, such as dust and soot, we're putting into our air locally and what is being blown in from outside our immediate region. For example, vehicle tailpipes emit nitrogen oxides, soot, and $CO_2$ as well as chemical toxins, such as benzene. Power plants release soot, nitrogen oxides, sulfur dioxides, and $CO_2$, among other pollutants. Factories, businesses, and residences also emit a variety of chemical compounds that pollute our air.

$CO_2$ is the most important greenhouse gas because there's more of it in the atmosphere than any of the others, but methane is the second most important greenhouse gas for causing climate change and ozone is the third most important. Nitrogen oxide and black soot are also important air pollutants that add to climate change. Interestingly, $CO_2$ was not initially considered an air pollutant because it is a normal component of our air, but we now know how damaging it is to the environment when there's too much of it.

In a warmer world, severely restricting the amount of pollutants we pump into the air we breathe every day will be even more critical. These air pollutants form another positive feedback loop, or snowball effect, that we frequently see with climate change: air pollutants cause climate change, then climate change causes air pollution to get worse, which causes more climate change and so on, causing an endless, worsening cycle.

Methane, which comes primarily from animal agriculture, is a strong greenhouse gas in its own right, but it is also a major contributor to the formation of ozone.[1] As food animals produce most methane, we'll address this topic more thoroughly in the chapter on food. Methane is also called "landfill gas" because it's released when leftover food and dead plants and animals decay and there's little or no oxygen available, which may occur at the bottom of a landfill. Carbon monoxide, which many people will recognize as being extremely deadly to breathe, also contributes to the formation of ozone and climate change.[2] Air pollutants actually harm us twice; they contribute to climate change while also causing harmful effects to the people and other living beings that breathe them.

## OZONE AND HEALTH

One of the most harmful air pollutants is ozone, the primary component of what we typically call "smog." (As an aside, this ozone is found at ground level but is made of the same stuff as the ozone you often hear about in our upper atmosphere as part of the "ozone hole." That upper-atmosphere ozone is actually good for us because it forms an atmospheric blanket that protects us from the sun's harmful ultraviolet rays. It's the same molecule in both places; whether it's causing us harm or protecting us simply depends on where the ozone is in relation to where we are. If it's at ground level where we can breathe it, it's bad. If it's in the upper atmosphere, it's good. What's more, ozone that is produced at ground level doesn't "live" long enough to make it up to the upper atmosphere to plug up the ozone hole, so ground-level ozone really has no redeeming qualities.) Ozone in smog is formed in the presence of heat and sunlight from nitrogen oxides and a variety of carbon-containing chemical fumes called *volatile organic compounds (VOCs)*. Some of these fumes come from natural sources, such as trees and forests, but in urban areas most come from the fumes that evaporate off paints, solvents, and gasoline. Those soft rubber gaskets that you see on gas pump nozzles are supposed to keep the gasoline fumes in your tank as you're filling up your vehicles instead of allowing the fumes to waft into the atmosphere to form smog.

With climate change, we expect hotter temperatures and plenty of sunshine. As a result, summertime ozone concentrations will increase in most regions. The warmer temperatures also will start earlier in the year, cause more hot days, and end later, effectively making summer last longer and causing more ozone formation. In a changing climate, summers in the United States are likely to have more frequent and intense high-ozone events.[3] One study of 50 cities in the eastern half of the United States projected an increase of 60 percent more days with ozone levels higher than the current health-based standard if climate change is allowed to proceed.[4]

Having more high-ozone days would be bad news because ozone is harmful to breathe and is already a problem in the United States and around the world. Ozone directly damages lung tissue in everyone who breathes it, even for short periods of time, although the body appears to repair the damage that occurs after a short time of exposure. Longer ozone exposure, though, can cause or worsen chronic lung diseases. Adults and children who are outside playing, exercising, or working when ozone concentrations are high may suffer from shortness of breath, coughing, or chest pain.

## WHO IS MOST VULNERABLE TO OZONE EFFECTS?

Because ozone damages lungs, people who have lung diseases, such as asthma, have a harder time when ozone concentrations are high. Under these conditions, they must take higher doses of their medicines to control their breathing and are more likely to end up in emergency rooms or be admitted to the hospital.

### Children

Asthma hits children especially hard. Currently, 9 percent of all American children have asthma. Although fewer children die from asthma now than was the case before 1999, asthma causes American children to miss almost 13 million days of school and has resulted in double the number of doctor visits during the last 10 years. The states with the highest percentages of children with asthma, according to the U.S. Centers for Disease Control, are Massachusetts, Hawaii, Oklahoma, Maryland, and Rhode Island. Asthma rates are even higher in Canada, where as many as one in five boys and one in six girls between the ages of 8 and 11 have asthma.

Not only does ozone make asthma worse in people who already have it, it has been shown to *cause* asthma. A group of scientists in California followed normal, healthy children and found that children who played three or more outdoor sports in towns with higher ozone levels were three times more likely to develop asthma than children who played outdoor sports in towns with lower ozone levels.[5] So asthma-causing ozone is a special concern, considering that climate change is causing ozone concentrations to increase.

Ozone is particularly damaging to children and babies because their lungs are not yet fully developed. Breathing ozone at an early age results in reduced lung capacity as an adult. Children also have more lung surface area for their weight, which means that they breathe more air for their weight than adults. That increases their exposure to any pollutants in the air. Children also spend more time outdoors than most adults, exposing them to more air pollution. Ozone concentrations are highest in the late afternoon and in the summer—times when children are most likely to be playing outdoors. Interestingly, breathing higher concentrations of ozone for several years may also predispose children to developing the kind of diabetes that requires insulin shots.[6]

Air pollution also harms fetuses growing inside women's wombs; ozone, carbon monoxide, and particulate matter are associated with higher rates of miscarriage, premature delivery, and lower-birth-weight infants.[7] It's not entirely clear which pollutants under what conditions are most responsible for causing these problems, but as air pollution likely causes harm to unborn babies, reducing the amounts of pollutants in the air—and preventing climate change—would help to protect these vulnerable members of our society.

## Other Vulnerable Populations

Other high-risk groups for air pollution include the elderly and anyone with heart or lung disease. During heat waves, air pollution—especially ozone—increases. The combination of high temperatures and bad air is particularly deadly. During the summer heat wave of 2003, when more than 45,000 people in western Europe perished, the highest ozone concentrations for the summer occurred when temperatures were highest and probably played a major role in the deaths of many people.[8,9] The vast majority of those heat wave victims were elderly.

Other research suggests that females may be more susceptible to the dangerous effects of ozone. In one study, mice were exposed to three hours of air containing a high dose of ozone and then infected with pneumonia. These mice died in higher proportions than mice that were exposed only to pneumonia but not ozone. However, the pneumonia infection killed more ozone-exposed female mice than males. For obvious reasons, the experiment can't be repeated in humans, but researchers wonder if air pollution, especially ozone, has a bigger effect on the immune systems of females than males.[10]

About a third of the U.S. population lives in areas with ozone concentrations that are already higher than the U.S. Environmental Protection Agency recommends. With that many people exposed to ozone, its negative effects go beyond lung damage. In addition to the suffering caused to individuals, there is a cost to society as well. Students miss school from asthma and other lung infections. More adult heart and lung disease results in lost income from missed work and higher medical care costs. And loss of life leads to fewer productive work years and income earned, as well as considerable sadness for loved ones left behind.

## PARTICULATE MATTER

Another major component of air pollution is *particulate matter*, the term given to a variety of tiny particles in the air, such as dust or soot. Soot, sometimes called black soot or black carbon, is a product of combustion and is released from power plants, especially those burning coal, as well as some engines, especially diesel engines. All particulates are dangerous to breathe, but *fine particulates* are the most dangerous. These tiny particles are small enough to penetrate deep into the lungs, and they frequently carry other toxins. Once they've arrived in the lungs, the particulates can result in respiratory symptoms, such as coughing or shortness of breath, as well as respiratory illnesses, such as bronchitis. The particulates can also aggravate asthma, decrease lung function, and cause premature death. Moreover, breathing particulate matter increases one's risk for suffering a heart attack.[11] Research has shown that children who live close to busy roads have more problems from particulate matter. Therefore, separating residential areas from heavy traffic areas would help to decrease children's—and everyone else's—exposure to these harmful pollutants.[12]

Particulate matter is also causing another major problem: new evidence shows that particulate matter carried from industrialized countries in the Northern Hemisphere to the Arctic on established wind currents, then deposited on the snow and ice, is partly responsible for causing the Arctic to melt so quickly. The dark-colored soot absorbs more of the Sun's energy and melts the ice and snow more quickly than the warmer air temperatures from global warming can do alone.[13] Helping industrializing countries like China and India use clean energy sources instead of coal, and helping to transfer technology to these countries to remove more of the black soot from their smokestacks, would help keep the Arctic frozen and the climate stabilized. This task is more manageable than the reduction of global greenhouse gas emissions, and it could be accomplished fairly quickly, buying some time to work on the bigger tasks of building an alternative energy infrastructure to take the place of the current fossil fuel system.

## FOREST FIRES AND BREATHING

One source of soot that is expected to increase with climate change is soot from forest fires, which are projected to be more common in a warmer world. The increase will be primarily from a combination of more drought conditions and big storms that generate more lightning.

Children, the elderly, and persons with heart and lung problems are especially affected and should avoid exposure to smoke if at all possible. Everyone, even healthy adults, should limit their exposure to smoke and should avoid physical activity outside when smoke is present.

Forest fires are already a big problem for health and well-being, particularly in the western United States. During the fall of 2007, more than 20 large fires burned in Montana and Idaho, producing thick clouds of smoke that occasionally spread across the Great Plains and even to the East Coast. In California, fires regularly threaten life and property, with thick clouds of smoke blanketing large areas during fire season.

In 1997 and 1998, fires raged through major forests on five continents. In Indonesia, fires severely damaged many large forests and blanketed the area with thick smoky haze for months. Researchers there found that up to 80 percent of the population suffered from such respiratory symptoms as coughing and shortness of breath. Persons who had respiratory illnesses prior to the fires were hit the hardest, with death rates in a respiratory hospital two to four times higher than occurred during the months before the fires. In 2006, Indonesia again experienced large fires that closed airports and drove away tourists, affecting the economic stability of the region. A stiff increase in deadly auto accidents occurred as a result of limited visibility when residents of Jakarta, Indonesia's capital and its largest city, fled the smoke in record numbers.

Smoke from large forest fires not only compromises the health of local communities but can travel great distances, affecting populations far away from the source. In 2002, Canada experienced large fires in Quebec province. The smoke from those fires was tracked all the way to Baltimore, Maryland, more than 700 miles (1127 km) away, where concentrations of fine particulates were 30 times higher than normal. Recently, researchers from Johns Hopkins Bloomberg School of Public Health determined that the higher concentration of fine particulates had caused increased hospitalizations for the elderly population in the 11 eastern U.S. states affected by the smoke.[14]

## DUST

Smoke is not the only air pollutant that doesn't respect international borders. Dust, laden with nitrates, sulfates, ozone, and other industrial toxins belching from China's busy smokestacks, blows clear across the Pacific Ocean to cause problems for those living on the West Coast of the United States. Warming temperatures combined with deforestation and overgrazing are changing more of China's land into deserts, fueling larger and more frequent dust storms. The dust storms are becoming more and more of a problem for China's residents, even in the capitol city of Beijing where residents apprehensively await the spring dust season. It's ironic that the production of goods has largely moved out of the United States and into China and southern Asia due to lower labor costs and less stringent environmental laws there. China's rapid industrialization has created inexpensive products for consumers all over the world but has added industrial pollutants to the air that are ending up back in the United States.

The Atlantic Ocean is experiencing its own problems with blowing dust from the ever-expanding deserts of northern Africa. Instead of industrial toxins, the African dust carries fungal spores that are deposited on coral beds in the Caribbean. The coral-killing fungus is devastating already stressed coral reefs, further jeopardizing their survival. Read the chapter on ecosystems for more information about how important coral reefs are to our health and well-being.

## OTHER AIR TOXINS

Other hazardous air pollutants, some regulated by existing legislation, have been implicated in climate change. The U.S. Clean Air Act amendments of 1990 listed 188 different chemicals as *hazardous air pollutants*. The U.S. Environmental Protection Agency is still developing emissions standards for these chemicals, many of which are found primarily inside the home. New products, such as furniture, construction materials, plastics, and paint, often release these hazardous air pollutants into the air for months to years—a process called *off-gassing*. Other products that are commonly used in some homes, such as pesticides and cleaning products, also release some of these hazardous air pollutants. Many of these products are volatile organic compounds that can mix with other chemicals to form ozone smog and potentially worsen climate change. More research is needed to determine how much these hazardous air pollutants contribute to climate change, but the toxicity of many of these chemicals to human health is often already known.

Most hazardous air pollutants are likely to be found outside our homes, though, and are emitted primarily by chemical manufacturing plants, refineries, waste incinerators, and other large industries as well as some smaller businesses like dry cleaners and paint and body shops. These outdoor air pollutants likely contribute to climate change, and the pollutants will only become more damaging as climate change unfolds. One group of researchers looked at 148 hazardous air pollutants in the state of Minnesota and found that 10 in particular occurred in concentrations high enough to potentially pose human health problems.[16] One of the compounds was benzene, a particularly toxic compound that may cause leukemia at higher doses, but it is not known whether the typical levels found in urban air could lead to this disease.[17] About half of the benzene in the atmosphere comes from gasoline, whereas the other half comes predominantly from industrial processes that use benzene. Warmer temperatures will likely lead to more benzene evaporating from gasoline into the air we breathe, and benzene is one of the many volatile organic compounds that contribute to ozone formation and climate change.

## POLLEN AND CLIMATE CHANGE

The warmer temperatures associated with climate change will also contribute to more pollen in the air by allowing some plants to thrive in areas where they may not have lived previously. Ragweed is one of these plants, and not only will warmer temperatures allow ragweed to expand its range, it also will grow more quickly and produce more pollen that could cause more severe allergic responses.[18] Ragweed pollen is a big problem for hay fever sufferers because many people are allergic to it and it causes strong allergic reactions. Hay fever can trigger asthma, and people who have asthma typically do worse during hay fever season. As a final blow to asthma sufferers, warmer temperatures and higher $CO_2$ concentrations will extend the hay fever season with its more prevalent and potent pollens.[19]

## WHO DECIDES HOW CLEAN OUR AIR WILL BE?

Given the array of air pollutants, the U.S. Clean Air Act of 1963, and subsequent amendments strengthening the act and tightening air pollution regulations, has been amazingly successful at improving our air quality. During the past 30 years in the United States, air pollution emissions have decreased by a third despite a growing population, greater economic activity, and a huge increase in vehicle miles traveled. But as technology continues to improve and scientists conduct more studies on the effects of air pollution, it has become obvious that air pollution causes more damage to human health than we previously knew. Climate change is guaranteed to make the quality of the air we breathe worse unless aggressive steps are taken to further limit air pollution emissions. Fortunately, improved technology also enables industry to do a better job of cleaning the pollutants coming out of factories' smokestacks and vehicles' tailpipes.

Regional, national, and international efforts to tighten air quality regulations and to provide local agencies additional funding for monitoring and enforcement will offer immediate benefits to our health as well as help to stabilize the climate.

Although $CO_2$ is the biggest problem for causing climate change because it's the most prevalent of the air pollutants, it can't just be "scrubbed" out of smokestack emissions like many other air pollutants. *Clean coal* is a term that was first used in the 1980s by the coal industry and the U.S. federal government to describe processes to remove sulfur, nitrogen, and mercury pollutants from coal-fired power plants. As the public and policy makers have become more aware of the role of $CO_2$ in climate change, the term has now been expanded by the coal industry to refer to a technology that is in the works to "capture" the $CO_2$ before it escapes to the atmosphere and "store" it somewhere safely underground. Part of this process, known as carbon capture and storage, already has been used on a small scale by the oil industry for many years. That industry purchases manufactured $CO_2$ and pumps it into the ground to force more oil out of wells. The technology to capture the $CO_2$ from power plant smoke stacks, where the $CO_2$ is relatively dilute, is not yet available in a large-scale or cost-effective way. Moreover, coal plants are not necessarily located adjacent to where the geologically appropriate underground storage sites are, so the $CO_2$ would need to be transported to these sites.

Experts say it will likely be 10 years or more before carbon capture technology is ready to be used on a commercial scale. But there are three main limitations to carbon capture and storage: (1) The added energy to run the coal gasification plants and compress the $CO_2$ before it can be injected into the ground consumes about 45 percent of the energy yielded by burning the coal in the first place. (2) Underground storage chambers must last thousands of years without leaking because leakage would be deadly for populations living close to the site and devastating for the world's climate. And (3) huge volumes of $CO_2$ would need to be stored. At current rates of coal burning, 12 cubic miles (50 km$^3$) of $CO_2$—a cube of gas that is 12 miles high, long, and wide—would have to be pumped into the Earth's crust every day.[15] Retrofitting older coal-burning power plants for carbon capture and storage is more difficult and expensive, so new coal-fired power plants should be built to be compatible with carbon capture and storage.

The fastest way to reduce the amount of air pollution and reduce $CO_2$ emissions, of course, is to stop burning fossil fuels and especially coal, which is the dirtiest of the traditional fossil fuels. If we are to stop global warming and prevent climate chaos, we absolutely must stop building coal-fired power plants unless we can capture and store all the $CO_2$ that these plants would otherwise release into the atmosphere. Because carbon capture and storage is not yet feasible, we simply need to burn less coal. When power plants are built, they are expected to stay in service for 30 to 50 years. Once a company has invested millions of dollars in building a new power plant, it is very difficult to get it to shut the plant down prematurely—for obvious reasons. That's why it's so important to prevent any further coal-fired power plants from being built—at least until the carbon capture and storage technology can be used.

## AIR QUALITY AND YOUR MENTAL HEALTH

All of this talk about air quality in light of climate change may make you anxious. Maybe it should. Research indicates people who are exposed to more air pollution are more likely to have heightened anxiety and also depression. People also perceive themselves as having less well-being overall when they are exposed to air pollution.[20]

Research indicates that people have more anxiety and tension when they live near industrial air pollutants too, and people who perceive their air quality is worse are more likely to be depressed.[21,22] Air pollution also seems to heighten people's concerns—including children's concerns—for their health and the health of their family members; this alone may increase worry and engender more stress in people's daily lives.[23]

Air pollution, as we've noted, also exacerbates asthma. Children and adolescents who experience asthma are at least twice as likely to be anxious as those who don't have this condition.[24] They also are almost twice as likely to be depressed or socially withdrawn, and they report that they experience more general psychological distress. When children with asthma miss school and other activities, they may be more likely to question their ability to do well in those settings.[25] For people older than 60 who have asthma, depression, more than anxiety, is more prevalent.[26]

Several studies also suggest that air pollution, including pollution associated with vehicles, may worsen or contribute to higher rates of schizophrenia, the severe mental health disorder in which people see, hear, or otherwise experience things that aren't really happening and have beliefs that are out of touch with reality.[27]

In this chapter, we've also discussed ozone and other pollutants that result from the burning of fossil fuels, whether from power plants, businesses, or vehicles. Although more research is needed, it appears that exposure to such toxicants in the environment is associated with a higher risk for learning disabilities in children.[28] When there are higher levels of ozone and related pollutants, more violence in families occurs, and there are more phone calls to the police for mental health emergencies.[29] There is also well-documented evidence that exposure to high levels of lead, mercury, and other heavy metals contributes to major learning and behavioral difficulties in children.[30]

There is one caveat in all of this research: no one has yet examined these mental health outcomes in relationship to variables explicitly associated with climate change because of the difficulty in doing so. It seems safe to say, though, that if one of the outcomes of climate chaos is poorer air quality, we're likely to have a lot more mental health problems as a result.

## SOLUTIONS

As toxic as the air may get with warmer temperatures, there is immediate payback for action. Reducing all forms of air pollution provides instant benefits to our health by reducing asthma, heart disease, and mental problems. In addition, because of the feedback loop we mentioned earlier in the chapter, cleaning the air is the most important thing we can do to slow global warming and avoid climate chaos. Remember, we have control over how much the climate changes and how chaotic it gets. If we take action now, we can stabilize the climate.

### Individual Solutions

To reduce your exposure to harmful air pollution:

- Limit the time you spend driving. The closer you are to traffic, the greater your exposure to air pollutants. Even being inside a car with the windows rolled up doesn't offer protection from the pollutants outside.
- Don't exercise outdoors in high-traffic areas during the late afternoon or evening when ozone concentrations are highest.
- If you have heart disease, do not exercise where you're likely to breathe in diesel exhaust because it could increase your risk of heart attack.
- On ozone alert days or high air pollution days, stay indoors with the windows closed, if possible. If you are outdoors, don't exercise.
- If you have asthma, work with your doctor to make sure your medicines keep your symptoms controlled. If you need to use your quick-relief inhaler—or rescue therapy—more than twice a week, talk with your doctor about changing your medicine routine to better control your asthma.

- Reduce indoor air pollution by avoiding incense, candles (especially scented ones), strong-smelling chemicals such as solvents, or cleaning products.
- When purchasing paints, varnishes, refinishing chemicals, and the like, choose the least toxic products and those with the least volatile organic compounds (VOCs). This might require a trip to a "green" home improvement store.
- When using these "volatile" products, make sure the room is well ventilated, preferably with a fan blowing the fumes away from you and toward an open window or door.
- Stay away from cigarette smoke, and keep infants and children away from secondhand smoke as much as possible. Don't allow any smoking in your home.
- Find out what's in your air. The Web site www.scorecard.org contains government-provided information about which pollutants businesses and industries are legally allowed to release into the air. You can enter your zip code and find out who is releasing what into your air. You might be surprised—and saddened. (You won't find ozone in this report because it isn't *released* as a pollutant. It is formed in the air from other pollutants that are released.)
- The American Lung Association creates annual State of the Air reports for every county in the United States that monitors ozone concentration. You can find the most recent information on the Web site at www.lungusa.org.

To reduce your contribution to the air pollution and climate change problem:

- The next time you buy a car, buy the most fuel-efficient car you can afford. If you currently drive a big car, seriously consider downsizing. If you're worried that you might need that extra space, power, or four-wheel drive sometimes, count up how many times a year you'll actually need them. With the price of gas getting higher and higher, it might be cheaper to plan to rent a larger or specialized vehicle occasionally. The rest of the time, you'll be saving a lot of money with lower gas bills, and you'll be helping to clean the air and prevent climate chaos. You can compare the fuel efficiency of different car makes and models at http://www.fueleconomy.gov/.
- Drive less, walk more.
- Make one weekly trip to run all your errands instead of many trips throughout the week.
- Ride a bike. Many towns have local bicycling groups that can help you plan the best routes and find riding partners.

- Use public transportation. Many towns don't invest in public transportation because they don't think their citizens will use it. Demand rapid, dependable, comfortable, safe, and convenient public transportation systems in your town.
- Try carpooling to work or activities. Start with one or two days per week if you're not sure how it will work for you. Most cities and some larger employers offer carpool registries that can help you find a match. Some businesses and cities offer bonuses for carpoolers, such as parking spots close to the workplace. Many cities offer guaranteed rides home for carpoolers and dedicated public transit riders in case of emergency. Most of these programs don't charge for the service, but they do require potential users to register to be eligible for the service.
- Working from home just one day per week reduces your work-related air pollution by 20 percent.
- On high ozone days, avoid driving and don't use paints or solvents.
- Avoid using gasoline-powered tools such as lawn mowers, leaf blowers, or snow blowers. These small engines can produce up to 11 times as much pollution as an automobile. Use people-powered tools, such as push mowers, if possible. Shovels and rakes provide the possibility of heart-healthy physical exercise and don't contribute to noise pollution as a bonus. But if you don't regularly engage in physical activity, shoveling heavy snow isn't the best way to start! If you're over 40 or have any heart or lung conditions, check with your doctor before starting an exercise program.
- Solar-powered machines are becoming more available but are still somewhat pricey. Electric-powered machines do not produce emissions themselves, but the production of electricity does. Depending on how much coal your utility company uses, switching to electric machines might result in a net reduction of emissions. If you must use a gasoline-powered machine, use the newest, least-polluting model you can afford. Emissions standards have steadily improved during the past 10 years and should continue to do so.
- Weatherize your home to reduce the amount of energy needed to heat and cool it. Your utility company and local home-improvement stores will have more specific information about how to do this. If you have limited income, many cities have programs to help defray or eliminate the cost of improving the heating and cooling efficiency of your home. Check with your city's housing authority to find out what's available in your area.
- If replacing older appliances, use Energy Star-rated models and buy the most efficient models you can afford. Refrigerators, air conditioners, and furnaces are the home appliances that use the most energy, and they have become far more efficient in recent years. Energy savings can often pay for the difference in price in just a few years.

- Clothes dryers are also energy intensive, but more efficient models are not yet available. Hang clothes to dry on outside lines or inside racks.
- Regular fireplaces and gas log fireplaces may provide nice ambiance, but they are horribly inefficient ways to heat a space, often pulling in more cold air than they heat. Both indoor and outdoor air pollution from these devices is usually substantial, and they should not be used. Newer, high-efficiency, airtight woodstoves, some burning agricultural products such as corn, can be more efficient than traditional furnaces. Significant differences in efficiency between products dictate that you do your research before deciding which one to buy.

## Community Solutions

In addition to making changes in your personal life, you can work with your community to make changes:

- Work with local and national organizations to pass legislation tightening regulations for how much air pollution power plants and industries can legally release into the air. As you work to pass legislation, remember that this is not just an environmental issue. Air pollution is a huge health issue. Get your local health professionals and health organizations involved in your efforts. Even health insurance companies should be interested in helping to pass legislation to reduce air pollution. After all, reducing asthma, hay fever, heart disease, and cancer lowers their costs. Getting the medical community involved was critical for passing the Healthy Air Act in Maryland in 2006, limiting sulfur, nitrogen, mercury, and $CO_2$ emissions.
- If you suspect there may be toxins in your air that aren't being adequately reported by their producers, special air-testing "buckets" can be used to check air samples. The Louisiana Bucket Brigade has been training communities in the proper use of specialized buckets for air monitoring for years. Their Web site is http://www.labucketbrigade.org.
- Urge your local policy makers to join a regional initiative, such as the ones now present in the Northeast, West, and Midwest, to cap and trade greenhouse gas emissions. This strategy has proved effective with other types of pollutants, and if the caps are set low enough they could also be effective for $CO_2$. Additional information about cap and trade systems can be found on the U.S. Environmental Protection Agency's Web site.
- Move major traffic conduits away from residential areas to reduce the harm from vehicle air pollution.
- Work with local policy makers to make your community more friendly to walkers. With obesity rates soaring in the United States, getting more

people, including children, to walk and bike makes good health sense in a variety of ways. About a quarter of all car trips are one mile or less, and one in six is shorter than a half-mile. More people would be willing to walk and ride a bike if it were safer to do so. A lot of suburbs and even some cities don't have sidewalks, forcing pedestrians to walk in the street. Newer cities and suburbs have been built especially for our car culture and are not pedestrian friendly. Adding bike lanes and sidewalks, closing some streets to vehicular traffic to encourage more pedestrian and bicycle use, and rejuvenating areas to include a variety of local shops and interesting streetscapes can all help reduce the number of miles people travel in their cars.

- Mobilize your neighborhood to identify neighbors who are especially vulnerable to air pollution due to age, heart, or lung conditions and check on them more frequently during ozone alert days or air-quality alert days.

## Regional, National, and International Solutions

Some policies will be more effective if they are made at the state or national level:

- Work with local chapters of national organizations to improve national air-quality standards. Keeping track of legislation is a full-time job requiring more time than many of us can spare. Many organizations that work on air pollution issues have paid staff who follow the complicated progress of legislation so you don't have to. If you sign up for their e-mail alert services, you'll be notified when legislation concerning an issue that interests you is being considered. You will also be told what you should do to make a difference in getting the legislation passed.
- To avoid dangerous climate change, vote for political candidates who will commit to improving air quality and reducing greenhouse gas emissions by at least 20 percent below 1990 levels by 2020 and by at least 80 percent below 1990 levels by 2050.
- Urge policy makers to do the following:
  - Build no new coal-fired power plants unless they use carbon capture and storage technology, which is not yet available.
  - Continue to increase vehicle fuel efficiency.
  - Reduce subsidies for the fossil fuel industry, which only encourages the continued use of fossil fuels.
  - Provide funding to improve public transportation systems.
  - Resist the urge to substitute nontraditional fossil fuels, such as highly polluting oil from oil sands or shale, to make up for declining supplies of

petroleum. (There will be more about this issue in the chapter on ecosystem health.)

- Create incentives and mandates to increase energy production from clean, renewable sources.
- Encourage research and development into new and improved renewable energy sources.
- Create incentives and mandates to improve the energy efficiency of all appliances and electronics.
- Work cooperatively with China and other rapidly industrializing countries to reduce their black soot pollution, thus keeping the Arctic cooler.
- Finally, cooperate with international entities to create and participate in binding treaties to reduce global greenhouse gas emissions.

# Chapter 5

# Water: Water, Water Everywhere or Neverthere

Maria is up early on yet another scorching morning trying to juggle getting ready for work with motivating her kids to prepare themselves for school. She has already read the story in the paper about the coal plant's evident effort to cover up its emissions and is trying to decide what, if anything, she should do about it. "I'm a doctor with much sicker elderly patients than usual," she says to herself. "And I'm the mother of a son with severe asthma. I have to do something about all this."

Just then, she hears the anchor on the local morning television news show say there's an important bulletin.

"We interrupt this program to notify you that the city council is planning to vote tonight on increasing local water-use restrictions. The city has completed its studies, which indicate that the McField Reservoir has only about two months of water left for public use if our drought conditions persist. We've also learned that the state has indicated that the Tacamara River's water level is too low to be readily tapped to supplement our water supply. In addition, area wells are running dry at alarming rates. More to come during our noon and 4 pm news shows."

Maria calls out to Moravia, who joins her in the kitchen.

"You rang?" he says, smiling broadly as he comes to her call. Maria frowns.

"This is too serious, Mo, this climate change. I just heard there are going to be even worse water restrictions. Can it be worse than that?" she questions, forcefully pointing to the totally parched yard outside the kitchen window. "And how are we going to manage with Max and his family?" She hears the anxiety in her voice, feels the discouragement in her face.

"What sort of restrictions?" Moravia asks, his smile long gone.

"How should I know?" Maria asks irritably. "I'm sorry, I'm sorry. I don't mean to snap. It's just that we're under a lot of pressure, Mo, and I need your help."

"What can I do?" Moravia asks imploringly. He also is frightened about the way the drought, the heat, the polluted air, and the fuel restrictions have taken their toll on his family—on him—and he's been using humor to avoid thinking about it.

Maria gets out a piece of paper to make a list. At the top she writes, "Do a rain dance that works" and, in an effort to indicate she still has a sense of humor too despite her fear, pushes it in front of Moravia before writing anything more. He reads the brief sentence and tries to smile, but he knows that dancing won't make a bit of difference to their increasing water woes.

## RISKS TO OUR WATER

Water is blue gold, the most fundamental of all human needs. We can survive for weeks without food but only a few days without water. In the United States, most of us don't think much about water. We turn the tap and out it comes, clean and plentiful. For many of us around the world, climate chaos will change that.

Climate change is expected to modify precipitation patterns on the planet. Places that tend to be dry now, such as the Mediterranean region, North Africa, the Middle East, southern Australia, and the southwest United States, are likely to get even drier, perhaps severely so. Equatorial areas and the far northern and far southern regions of the globe are likely to become wetter overall. Practically all areas will experience greater variability in precipitation. Even places expected to get wetter may experience heavier rains falling on fewer days with longer dry spells in between and more inconsistency from season to season and from year to year.[1] This pattern may mean that less water is available for our consumption despite the heavier rains.

As much as we take water for granted here in the United States, most of us are aware that water is not so plentiful elsewhere in the world. Demand for water has tripled during the past 50 years, and currently a half billion people live in a water-stressed country. By 2025, that number is expected to increase to about three billion.[2] Those conditions exist without any effects from climate change. That increase simply indicates that water resources are becoming scarcer primarily due to their overuse and poor management. The amount of fresh water available on Earth does not increase, but the number of people wanting to use that water does—along with the amount of water they wish to use. The problem is further exacerbated by fresh water sources, especially rivers and lakes, becoming increasingly polluted and no longer available for use.

## HOW WE USE WATER

A surprising 52 percent of the fresh water we use in the United States is used to produce electricity. Once it cools our power plants, that water is generally returned to surface water sources, such as lakes and streams, so it can be reused for other purposes. If we exclude electricity production, 64 percent of our fresh water irrigates our crops; 25 percent is used residentially and commercially; about 6 percent is used in industry and mining; and smaller amounts are used for livestock, aquaculture, and other miscellaneous needs.[3]

The vast majority of the available fresh water on the planet—about 70 percent—is used for agriculture. In some countries like India, however, almost all of the fresh water goes to agriculture. Not all agricultural products require the same amount of water, but invariably most of the things we consume daily, including our food, require large amounts of water to produce or manufacture. Table 5.1 gives you an idea of how much water is required to make a variety of products. The United Nations Environment Programme projects that domestic and industrial uses will continue to increase, particularly in the developing world, and agricultural

Table 5.1. Amount of Water Required to Make Various Foodstuffs and Products

| Product | Gallons of Water Required |
| --- | --- |
| Office paper, 10 sheets | 1 |
| Orange juice, 1 glass | 3 |
| Crude oil, refine 1 gallon | 10 |
| Egg, 1 | 40 |
| Flour, 1 pound | 75 |
| Milk, 1 glass | 100 |
| Sunday newspaper | 280 |
| Rice, 1 pound | 560 |
| Beef, 1 pound | 2,500 |
| Aluminum, 1 pound | 1,000 |
| Automobile | 100,000 |

Source: U.S. Environmental Protection Agency, United Nations Environment Programme, U.S. Geological Survey, and Environmental Defense.

use also will increase. This combination could lead to conflict among the many users of this limited vital resource.[4]

The amounts of water needed to produce various products might surprise you. To produce beef, for example, a cow consumes grains and other plant matter for at least two years before being slaughtered. Cows, as you'll see in the food chapter, are not the most efficient animals when it comes to turning grain into meat. The greatest amount of water used in the production of meat is to grow the grain to feed the cow, but the cow also requires water to drink, the slaughtering process uses water, and transportation of the meat takes water too. This water use all adds up.

## WHERE OUR WATER COMES FROM

Our water supply comes from different places, partly depending on where we live. On the U.S. East Coast, much of the water supply comes from surface waters, whereas most of the Midwest gets its water supply from a combination of surface waters and well water. The well water comes from underground aquifers such as the Ogallala Aquifer. This is an ancient or "fossil" water supply, as little, if any, rainfall works its way into the aquifer to replenish the water we remove from the aquifer. When's it's gone, its gone. And it's going pretty fast.

Much of the farm and ranch lands of the eastern portions of Colorado and New Mexico, as well as the High Plains states of Nebraska, Kansas, Oklahoma, and western Texas, are irrigated using Ogallala water. At present rates of withdrawal, parts of the Ogallala Aquifer water will be available for irrigation for only another 10 to 20 years, although some areas should still be able to produce some water for irrigation for another 50 years.[5] Most of the areas currently drawing water from the aquifer do not receive enough rain to grow crops without irrigation, and there are few other sources of irrigation water available. Nonetheless counties and states are now taking steps to use the water more slowly.

On the West Coast, the greater Los Angeles area, with its population of more than 17 million people, "arranged" more than a century ago to get water from the Owens River that drains runoff from the Sierra Nevada Mountains. Although there continues to be some animosity between the inhabitants of the Owens Valley and the Los Angeles Basin about the manner in which the water was acquired, without that water the area could not have developed into the metropolis that it is now. About one-third of California's water supply comes from melting snow-pack along the 400-mile-long Sierra Nevada Mountains. The area also receives water from the Colorado River, from the northern part of the state, and from underground aquifers that have declining water reserves. The San Joaquin Valley in California provides much of the nation's food supply. That food could not be grown without water for irrigation. Although farmers have gotten better at growing more food with less water, they're still in danger of not having sufficient water to grow their crops. As we'll discuss later, climate change will put much of California's water supply at risk.

The desert Southwest, especially Arizona and New Mexico, gets about half of its water from melting snow in the Rocky Mountains and the other half from deep wells. Water tables in parts of Arizona have dropped by more than 500 feet. Taking water from deep beneath the surface of the Earth causes several problems. Not only is the water being depleted much faster than it can be replenished, causing concern about future water supplies, but water has mass. If the mass is removed, it leaves behind spaces in the ground. As the ground on top falls in to fill up the spaces, the land moves or "subsides." This subsidence has been so extensive in Arizona, for example, that some areas around the Phoenix metropolitan area have sunk five feet or more, causing building foundations and pipes to break. Areas around Eloy, Arizona, in the south-central area of the state, have sunk as much as 15 feet.[6] The desert Southwest is already facing water shortages. Climate change will further compromise the water supplies for this area as these dry areas get drier.

## HOW MUCH WATER WE NEED

The World Health Organization reports that a person needs about five gallons of water per day to meet the most basic needs of drinking, cooking, and very limited washing. To put this into perspective, more than a billion people lack access to clean water, and these people must get by on five quarts of water per day—the absolute minimum amount of water that an average adult must consume to stay alive. (To make it worse, that water is often contaminated with pollutants.[7]) That's less than 500 gallons a year! In contrast, each American uses an average of 70 gallons daily inside the house. Total monthly water usage for an average American household with a family of four is well over 10,000 gallons. Every day dripping faucets in rich countries lose more water than is available to about one-sixth of the world's population.[8]

In addition to having enough water to drink and cook our food, many of the practices we rely on to keep us healthy also involve having an adequate supply of clean water. Washing our hands after every trip to the bathroom, cleaning dishes, bathing, and washing our clothes are all important for keeping germs in check and staying healthy. Infants and children are especially susceptible to diseases carried by polluted water, and around the world 1.8 million children die each year—almost 5,000 every day—from unclean water and poor sanitation.[7]

## DROUGHTS AFFECT HEALTH

Lack of water also presents us with life-harming risks, and climate change will also contribute to the problem of droughts. Globally, the most severe health effect of an extended drought is crop failure leading to famine, as is occurring in many places in Africa. According to Ban Ki-moon, Secretary General of the United Nations, extended drought that is at least partially caused by climate change has played a role in the deadly conflict in the Darfur region of Sudan. Competition for scarce water originally helped to fuel the tension between Arab nomadic herders and the primarily African farmers there.[9]

Here in the United States, droughts have not caused famines, but water managers are very concerned about water supplies running short or becoming completely depleted. Water levels in the Great Lakes are far below normal, many regions of Florida have nearly tapped out their groundwater supply, the city of Atlanta in the normally damp Southeast instituted water restrictions when its reservoirs hit all-time lows, and Lake Powell on the Utah-Arizona border is almost two-thirds below normal levels. Scientists say the prolonged drought in the Southwest may be the new norm. Around the world, water shortages are growing.

## DROUGHTS AND INFECTIOUS DISEASE

In addition to the enormous problems droughts create for our daily consumption and food production, they also can lead to an increased risk of infectious disease. As the remaining water supplies shrink, amounts of contaminants, such as toxins and chemicals, and the number of microorganisms, including the bacteria, viruses, and parasites that cause disease, can all become more concentrated.

The tale of West Nile virus is illustrative. The mosquitoes that could carry West Nile virus had been living quite happily in New York for years before the virus arrived in 2001. At that time, New York had been suffering through a severe drought for the third year in a row. During times of drought, when fewer sources of surface water, such as lakes, ponds, and puddles, exist, wildlife are forced to congregate around the remaining water sources. That makes it easier for a biting insect, in this case a mosquito, to move from one host to the next, biting, taking a blood meal, and then moving on to another host nearby. If the mosquito is infected with West Nile virus, it passes that virus on to the animal or bird as it feeds on its blood. That animal or bird then becomes infected and unwittingly infects the next mosquito that bites it. In this way, droughts actually make it easier for a biting insect that carries the virus to be a more efficient spreader of disease. We'll discuss the impact that West Nile virus has had on the human population in the chapter on infectious disease.

Although no single weather event can be linked to climate change, more frequent and severe droughts are projected to occur in a warmer world, so the drought conditions in New York and elsewhere are consistent with what we expect from climate change. Although the virus arrived in the United States due to globalization, climate change likely contributed to its rapid and efficient spread.

## DROUGHTS AND FIRES

In addition to causing an increased risk of infectious diseases, droughts also increase the risk of forest and brush fires. In Greece, the summer of 2007 brought searing heat with temperatures in excess of 107°F (41.7°C), prolonged drought, and more than 3,000 fires. Despite the mobilization of 6,000 soldiers and fleets of water-dumping aircraft from other nations, fire still killed 65 people and charred entire villages and almost a half-million acres, including forests, brush, farmland, and olive groves.

Researchers have documented that warmer temperatures and earlier spring melt from climate change are largely responsible for the increase in western U.S. forest fires since the mid-1980s.[10] In 2006, drought conditions caused California to lose more than three-quarters of a million acres, 400 structures, and nine lives to forest fires. In 2007, California again experienced numerous fires, charring more than half a million acres, destroying more than 1,600 homes, requiring the rapid evacuation of more than a million people from their homes, and causing at least 14 deaths. Elsewhere in the western United States, more than 5 million acres burned in 2007. In the previous chapter on air quality, we talked about how the smoke from the fires can cause heart and lung problems, especially for the elderly.

Anyone who ever listened to Smoky the Bear knows that the drier a forest is, the more careful everyone needs to be with their cigarettes and campfires. Something you may not know, though, is that forest fires actually increase the risk of drought in several ways. Large forest fires can influence weather patterns, creating their own high-pressure system that drives away clouds and moisture. Massive deforestation of the Amazon rain forest, largely through burning, has resulted in drier conditions over part of the forest, leading to more forest fires. Moreover, once an area has burned, there are no more plants alive to absorb moisture into their roots, hold the soil in place, and allow the soil itself to hold more moisture. Without plants, more of the rain that falls on that land becomes runoff water, washing into streams and rivers and carrying silt and soil with it. The result is that it's much harder for trees to get a foothold and grow. Scientists believe that if current trends continue, 30 percent of the Amazon rain forest will be gone by 2050.[11]

Mudslides are a deadly side effect of drought and fires. With the onset of winter rains that put out the fires, California residents know that mudslides will follow because the fires have removed the vegetation that holds the soil in place, especially along the many steep canyon walls. So climate change will cause more droughts; droughts lead to forest fires; land without plants allows mudslides and contributes to more droughts; and so on.

## FLOODS AFFECT HEALTH

Climate change won't only contribute to droughts. It also will be a force behind floods as it pushes more moisture into the atmosphere and engenders stronger storms as a result. Floods are the most common natural disaster worldwide, causing local and sometimes regional devastation that harms thousands of people. Climate-related floods can result from heavy rain, causing lakes, rivers, and reservoirs to overflow; fierce storms or hurricanes that cause damage that leads to flooding; or storm surges. The frequency and intensity of floods are expected to increase as a result of climate change. We'll discuss the many health effects of floods in the next chapter on cataclysmic events.

## CLIMATE CHANGE AND WATER AVAILABILITY

To understand how climate change will affect the availability of water, it's helpful to understand a bit about the hydrological cycle—the way in which water moves from the oceans to the atmosphere to the soil and back to the oceans. Warm air over the oceans absorbs water to form clouds. The clouds then move on established air currents, and a variety of factors influence how and when the water from the clouds falls as rain to the ground. Some of the rain runs off into rivers and streams and flows directly back to the sea. Some rain soaks into the ground, where it is taken up by plant roots for use in the plants' metabolic processes and then released from the leaves into the air. And some rain soaks into the ground and recharges aquifers. The moisture in the air re-forms into clouds that carry the moisture farther inland. It will eventually fall again as rain or snow, some of it soaking into the ground again and some of it running off into rivers and streams and returning to the oceans. In general, warmer air holds more moisture. With the warming temperatures that accompany climate change, this means that more moisture will be absorbed from the oceans into the atmosphere, and therefore overall global precipitation will increase. But the result will not be uniform; some areas will get more rain, and some will get less.

From this accurate but simplified description, it becomes obvious that plants play an integral role in "moving" water from the oceans inland. In China, for example, where major deforestation has occurred in some regions, inland areas are becoming drier as a result. Bare or sparsely vegetated ground leads to greater runoff, greater erosion, and speedier moisture evaporation. This partly explains why places that have histori-cally been dry will likely get drier in a warmer world. The Chinese gov-ernment is now working to reforest large parts of China to combat the droughts that have gripped these regions.

As paradoxical as it sounds, flooding often leads to less available fresh water, not more. When rain comes in large quantities during a short time, there's less time for the water to soak into the ground, and more of it becomes runoff into rivers and the sea. That water becomes "lost" for the purpose of providing fresh water for residences and farms. Figure 5.1 shows scientists' projections of changes in rainfall in the United States in 2100 if we do not reduce greenhouse gases and if climate change is allowed to continue. Climate change really means changing rainfall pat-terns that could become chaotic if the climate is not stabilized.

## MELTING SNOWPACK

With warmer temperatures overall—meaning spring will come earlier, fall will last longer, and winter will be shorter—more of the precipitation that falls during the colder months will be rain instead of snow. Although some people might initially rejoice that they won't have to shovel as much snow during the winter, the implications for water availability are sobering. Snow in the mountains accumulates all winter and then begins to melt in the spring, providing a steady water supply through the late spring and summer when rains are typically scarce and crops need the most water. If more pre-cipitation falls as rain, it doesn't build up into a snowpack. With tempera-tures climbing earlier in spring, the snowpack that does form will melt more quickly, potentially causing floods. Spring snowpack in the Cascade

Mountains in Oregon and Washington, for example, could drop by as much as 60 percent, reducing summer stream flows by 20 to 50 percent.[12]

Many parts of the country and world rely on snowmelt for their water supply. The U.S. Southwest, as we've mentioned, gets most of its water supply from the melting snowpack in the Rocky Mountains, but even states in the Midwest get much of their water from melting snowpack in the Rockies. The Arkansas River, for example, starts in the Rocky Mountains and supplies water to cities and farms across the plains before emptying into the Mississippi River in its namesake state.

## MELTING GLACIERS

Many major population areas around the world also rely on the slow, steady melt of high mountain glaciers to provide a reliable water source. The Himalayas provide water for much of India, Pakistan, Bangladesh, and western China. As those glaciers melt more quickly, the areas downstream will have plenty of water and could even experience flooding in the next several decades. The glaciers hold *fossil water*, however—water

## Projected Annual Precipitation Changes for 2091-2100

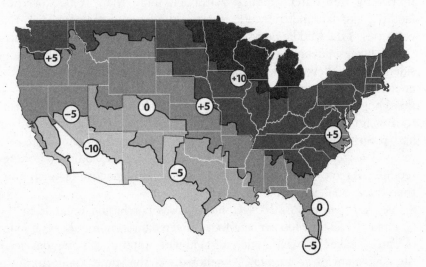

**Figure 5.1** This map shows the changes in the percentage of precipitation relative to 1971–2000 averages for the United States if we do not reduce greenhouse gas emissions. Source: JL Weiss, The University of Arizona, with data from Hoerling & Eischeid NOAA ESRL.

that is not replaceable in a human time frame. Once those glaciers have melted, releasing their water to the sea, that water is gone. Many large cities in Europe that depend on melting glaciers in the Alps, communities in South America that depend on the many melting glaciers of the Andes, and sprawling cities that depend on the Himalayas' glaciers— altogether about a billion people—will face massive water shortages. This presents a unique psychological and communication challenge because it's hard to persuade people that they need to conserve water when there is no current shortage and, in fact, there is a surplus. However, the glaciers of the Andes are expected to disappear in as little as 15 years, causing water shortages for 60 percent of Peruvians and electricity shortages for the 40 percent who currently get their electricity from hydroelectric plants using glacier-melt rivers.[11,13]

As you can see, water supplies and potential water scarcity are extremely dependent on climate. A study using computer modeling indicates that one third of Earth's land surface will be at risk for extreme drought by 2100 compared to the 1 percent that is currently at risk for extreme drought.[14] With looming water shortages, desalination has been suggested as an easy solution. We'll address the pros and cons of desalination next.

## DESALINATION

Desalination, the removal of salt from seawater, might be an option for increasing freshwater supplies. Although more than 10,000 of these facilities exist around the world, most of them are in the petroleum-rich countries of the Middle East because the water they produce is very costly.

The biggest advantage of desalination is that seawater generally is considered "free." Beyond that, however, there are several disadvantages, the greatest being the energy requirements associated with this process. It takes huge amounts of electricity to remove salt from seawater so it's safe for human consumption. Of the two primary methods used, distillation and reverse osmosis, distillation requires heating the water and thus requires more energy. Even with reverse osmosis, the additional energy required to remove the salt results in the final product costing much more than traditional water sources.

As a comparison, in 2004 California was purchasing water from the Colorado River for $460 per acre-foot delivered (an acre-foot is the amount of water it takes to cover an acre of land with water that is one foot deep, the equivalent of about 325,000 gallons). At that time, California estimated that using water that had been desalinated by the reverse osmosis method would cost up to $1,500 per acre-foot. If a municipality must pay three times more for its water, other services will likely need to be scaled back or customers' water bills will have to be raised to cover the added cost. If the price of electricity increases, the price of desalinating water will increase accordingly. California estimates that 13 megawatts of electricity (the average amount required to power 4,000 homes) are needed to produce 1 million gallons of desalinated water, which would serve about 100 U.S. homes for 1 month.[15] Because we're already using all the electricity we're producing, getting more of our water from desalination facilities would require building many new power plants.

Other potential disadvantages to desalination are that it's only feasible on the coast. Transporting water inland increases the cost exponentially. There is also potential for the destruction of coastal habitat because these massive plants are situated at the water's edge for ease of access to seawater. If brackish water is used instead of seawater, less electricity is needed because there's less salt to remove, but there's greater potential for coastal habitat destruction if the source water is taken from more inland bays, estuaries, or wetland areas. As you'll see in the next chapter, positioning desalination plants at the water's edge puts the plants themselves at risk of flooding from a rise in sea level or destruction from storms. In addition to all the economic costs, however, there is the additional cost of the electricity producing added greenhouse gases, which contribute to global warming, which causes more droughts or storms with rapid runoff, which encourages more desalination. This is yet another of those positive feedback loops, which aren't really positive at all, that we've talked about in this book.

Just so you know, the process used to remove salt from water can also be used to process wastewater into pure, clean, safe drinking water. Once you get past the "yuck factor," using wastewater may make more sense for many regions than desalination . . . except for those high energy costs. This process is already under way in several areas of the world, including the United States.

## BOTTLED WATER

As we discuss the potential for increased water scarcity and the energy required for water supplies, the relatively new issue of bottled water is instructive. Many people have the sense that bottled water is purer or safer than tap water. In the United States, bottled water is now subject to safety regulations similar to municipal water systems. But the U.S. Food and Drug Administration, the agency charged with setting and enforcing regulations for bottled water, reports that this product is no safer than tap water.[16] In

addition, the energy required to produce plastic bottles, which use petroleum as a starting ingredient, and to transport billions of bottles of water all
over the country and the world, is staggering. Moreover, fewer than 14 percent of those plastic bottles in the United States are recycled. The Earth
Policy Institute reports that global consumption of bottled water now
exceeds 41 billion gallons. The United States, as the world's largest single
consumer, drinks more than 7 billion gallons of bottled water each year—
requiring 17 million barrels of oil just to make the required 29 billion plastic bottles. When you add in the energy for pumping, processing,
transportation, and refrigeration, the total comes to 50 million barrels of oil
per year just to meet America's thirst for bottled water![17]

At a time when global supplies of crude oil—much less water—are
becoming ever more dear, we need to rethink the way we use both of
these declining resources. Mexico and China are the second and third
largest consumers of bottled water. As their economies provide additional
disposable income to their citizens, their consumption of bottled water
and the crude oil needed to produce it also will grow.

## WATER CONSERVATION—MORE THAN
## JUST PERSONAL VIRTUE

In places with previously plentiful supplies of water, no one thought
much about trying to conserve this resource. The effects of climate
change, however, combined with population growth and runaway development, threaten water supplies all over the world, including those of
industrialized countries. Using less water should be the first goal for
everyone, everywhere. Delivering fresh, clean, safe water to your tap
requires energy; heating the water for use in your home requires energy;
and processing the wastewater—even if it's only to a level that is less
damaging to discharge into our waterways—requires energy. Currently,
that energy supply produces greenhouse gases that fuel climate change.
We've included some water conservation tips in the solutions section at
the end of the chapter. Water conservation, which usually leads to lower
water bills, is one of those situations in which everyone benefits.

## WATER SCARCITY, CONSERVATION, AND MENTAL HEALTH

With the importance of our water supply to our existence, our concerns
about the effects of climate change on this resource, and evidence that
adequate water resources are a flash point for human conflict, it would

seem prudent to conserve our precious water resources and prepare for problems involving water.[18-20] Some people and places are doing just that, but water conservation behavior is complex.

Research indicates, for instance, that people who perceive water as an unlimited and disposable resource are more likely to consume more of it than people who recognize both the limits of our water resources and our tendency to exploit natural resources without heed for the repercussions.[21] This is similar to the finding that people who are self-interested tend to consume more water than people who are concerned about the environment.[22] Other factors that play into conservation behavior include our beliefs, community norms, and access to accurate, clear information about water availability.[23] If people aren't going to take the initiative to conserve water, enforcing conservation through careful water metering or fines has been shown to be an effective tool in shaping people's water conservation actions.[21,24] In regard to polluted water, people who understand the importance of their water resources and realize that they're in poor shape are more willing to clean them up.[25] Yet, even when we express strong support for water conservation, our actual engagement in water conservation activities often lags behind our professed concern.[26]

Given this gap between our concern and our water conservation efforts, there is some anecdotal evidence that a lack of sufficient clean water can lead to psychological distress.[27] Despite the limited research, one study found that people in a drought-plagued region of Brazil had much higher rates of anxiety and general emotional distress than people who lived in a similar area without drought.[28] Another study found youths in rural Australia were aware of the stress a persistent drought had on them and their families, even though they reported that they were coping with it well.[29]

Finally, other research examined whether mild dehydration affects people's thinking and abilities to act, and although there was no evidence that such people were impaired, mildly dehydrated people did say that they were more tired, less alert and able to concentrate, and needed to make more effort to accomplish certain tasks.[30,31]

Despite the scant evidence about how water shortages affect us, it's clear that droughts and related water problems do focus people's attention on these crises and their implications—even though people might not understand their role in creating and preventing these problems.[32] We have work to do then to connect our understanding of the existence of climate-induced water woes to what we can do to prevent the harm that shortages of water cause.

# SOLUTIONS

## Individual Solutions

Here are some ways that you can improve the safety of the water you consume and ways that you can conserve water.

- Take the time to learn about water resources in your community, whether these resources are at risk, and what you can do to prevent harm from potential drought or pollution.
- Educate your family, friends, neighbors, and coworkers about the need to conserve water and some of the ways they can do so.
- In the United States, municipal water systems are required to send consumers annual reports of water quality. Look at these reports carefully and ask questions about anything you don't understand or that looks troublesome.
- If your tap water looks discolored or has an odor, don't use it and contact your local water authority immediately.
- During power outages or after big storms, listen to the advice of public authorities about the safety of tap water. You may need to boil the water until water treatment plants are up and running and the system has been adequately flushed.
- When in doubt, boil your water. To be safe, bring the water to a rolling boil for one full minute. If you live above 6,500 feet (2000 m) elevation, boil for a full three minutes.
- Replace older appliances with newer, water-conserving appliances. See Table 5.2 for a comparison of how much water can be saved by switching.

Table 5.2. Household Water Use and Ways to Conserve

| Appliance | Older Models Use | Newer, Conserving Models Use |
|---|---|---|
| Shower | 5 to 8 gal/min | 1.6 to 2.5 gal/min |
| Toilet | 3.5 to 5 gal/flush | 1.6 gal/flush |
| Washing machine | 32 to 50 gal/load | 18 to 24 gal/load |
| Dishwasher | 13 to 25 gal/load | 9 to 11 gal/load |
| Sink faucets | 4 gal/min | 1 to 2.75 gal/min with aerator |
| Leaky faucet | 1 drip/second wastes 9 gallons/day | 0 when leak is fixed! |

Data from *Sustainability of Semi-Arid Hydrology and Riparian Areas*, University of Arizona Cooperative Extension (http://www.sahra.arizona.edu/programs/water_cons/home/meter.htm).

- Replace water-guzzling lawns with native vegetation that requires little to no additional watering (and no fossil fuels are required for mowing).
- Be aware of how much water you use and try to reduce the amounts. The following Web sites have many good ideas for ways to conserve water, including low-flow fixtures, inside and outside.
  - http://www.wateruseitwisely.com/
  - http://www.fema.gov/areyouready/appendix_a.shtm
  - http://www.waterinfo.org/conservation-tips
- Avoid using bottled water. If you don't like the way your tap water tastes, filter it. And reuse your water containers, making sure you allow them to dry completely between uses to avoid mold.
- Eat less meat, especially beef, because beef requires more water per calorie to produce than other foods.

## Community Solutions

Working with your community, you can have an impact on the safety and conservation of your water sources.

- Make sure zoning laws require all new construction or major remodeling jobs include mandatory installation of water-conserving devices.
- Modify zoning laws to allow reuse of "gray water" (it comes out of the sink, tub, and washing-machine drains) for irrigation and landscape watering.
- Find out where the watershed for your water source is located and make sure it is protected from development and pollution.
- Encourage water pricing that motivates conservation. One way to do this is to progressively increase the price per unit of water with increased consumption (i.e., $20 for the first 1,000 gallons, $30 for the next 1,000 gallons, and so forth).
- Motivate community leaders and educators to widely promote water conservation and cleanliness and help make conservation a community norm.
- If you live in an agricultural area, encourage your policy makers to create incentives for agricultural consumers to install equipment and technology that allows them to use water more efficiently.

# Chapter 6

## Cataclysmic Events:
## Pounding People and the Planet

While Maria and Moravia are trying to figure out how they'll cope with the latest water restrictions in light of the six new family members and their pets who are coming to live with them, Max is getting ready to drive his family away from his worst nightmare. He hopes the distance will help ease the pain of years of mounting losses in the one place he had come to dearly love. Maybe in a new place, he thinks, he will be able to sleep through the night again, eat without experiencing indigestion, and work without distraction.

His family had begun packing fragile items and important belongings long before the latest hurricane, Carl, started forming off the coast of Africa. Last year, crashing waves and wind nearly destroyed the family's house and land during the largest spate of major hurricanes in recorded history. As a result, Max's wife Sula said they needed to begin looking for another place to live. She quietly and persistently nudged her family to begin the arduous task of determining what to take with them to their new life, wherever that would be, soon. While Sula planned, Max buried himself in his work . . . until the media showed just how massive Carl was becoming. Just days away now, this hurricane will, he knows, be the end of his family's once wondrous coastal life.

After packing their two SUVs and a trailer with as many of their belongings as they could cram into them in 24 hours, Max surveys his property and the sea one more time. His house, with its blue tarps on the roof, cracked walls, and broken foundation, doesn't stir much in him anymore. It had been a grand villa, by all appearances, but now it is just a structure to him. The sea, though, remains his passion. He loved to sail on it before the storms destroyed his classic sloop several years ago, and even now he has continued to adore being close to its seething, calming, beckoning waters. Now, as he moves along the spot where his narrowing property meets the water, churning with the latest approaching storm, he can see how the sea has angrily gobbled up swathes of his land, clawing ever closer to his home. The water has crept higher, consuming the land, making his well water saltier year by year. He knows all this from real experience, from his family's growing stress, from the latest reports about climate change. But now, coupled with another storm that yet again could be "the one," Max realizes that he no longer has the fight in him to tackle these problems.

"I see that you're taking all of this away from me." he says. Max hears himself softly talking to the water as the gray waves smack against the retaining wall that is the final barrier between his house and the sea, "You've been doing it for years. I know I should have listened long ago when I could have done something other than throw a few little walls in your way. We should have listened to you. . . ."

He blows the raging sea an awkward kiss, feeling silly as he does so, and walks to his car that will take him away forever. Close behind him, the swelling waves crash against the wall again and again.

## A CAVALCADE OF HARM

Stronger hurricanes, heavy rains, the rising sea level, searing heat waves, droughts, forest fires, and more will be among the catastrophes that come with climate change and, put simply, they're going to harm many of us. We've already discussed many of these high-damage events, but in this chapter we will give you a broader understanding of their implications for our health and well-being.

Many of these events occur together like links in a chain. Hurricane Katrina, which certainly harmed thousands of Gulf Coast residents and awakened the United States to the devastation of a cataclysmic natural event, not only produced high winds and rains. It also combined with flooding, storm surge, erosion, and freshwater contamination to force tens of thousands to flee and make much of the coast uninhabitable.

Let's begin to examine these cataclysmic events with a look at how floods affect our health. Flooding already accounts for about 40 percent of the world's natural disasters and half of the deaths from them.[1] After addressing other major events associated with climate change, we'll attend to the science of a sea level rise and hurricanes, two of the more complicated climate-change events we're likely to face.

## FLOODS AND INUNDATIONS

When Hurricane Katrina slammed into the Gulf Coast in 2005, it wasn't her high winds that caused the most damage. It was the flooding. Floods can cause death and disease from drowning, infectious diseases, mold, and contaminated water supplies, and they can have mental health repercussions. Floods also can contribute to malnutrition and starvation when crops are damaged and transportation is interrupted. All the research indicates that climate change will bring on conditions that will enhance the size and scope of these floods.

It probably comes as no surprise that people are injured and killed during floods. During Hurricane Katrina and the flooding that occurred after the levees broke, 1,800 people lost their lives, primarily from drowning. Injuries and deaths can also occur as residents attempt to rescue themselves and their belongings and when they return to their homes to clean up and repair the damage.

Floods can result from fresh water, such as the heavy rains that fell on the Gulf Coast during Hurricane Katrina, from rivers overflowing their banks, from levees collapsing, or from dams giving way. Floods also can result when a rising sea level inundates land with salt water or from the storm surge that occurs during big storms. We'll get to storm surge in a moment.

Despite the common belief that floods happen mostly in poor countries, national wealth and industrialization do not necessarily offer protection from floods. During the summer of 2007, heavy rains left a third of a million people in southern England without fresh water and thousands seeking refuge in Red Cross shelters. On the other hand, developing countries may struggle much more because they have fewer resources to use for recovery, as happened in Mumbai, India, in 2005 where three feet (1 meter) of rain fell in four hours. Because that rain coincided with a high tide, further hampering the city's storm drainage capability, at least 3 million people were exposed to severe flooding. Although there were only 100 immediate deaths from drowning or injury during that catastrophe, more than 150,000 people were treated later for flood-related illnesses.[2]

Even if flood victims survive the immediate danger of the flood, they're still at risk for health problems. Flood survivors have higher rates of physical illnesses, such as diabetes, high blood pressure, and heart disease. Two studies in the United Kingdom found a 50 percent increase in deaths from these sorts of causes in flood survivors during the year after they had experienced a flood.[3] In the United States, high blood pressure rose by 35 percent in affected Mississippi families after Hurricane Katrina, and half of the parents and 40 percent of the children living in Federal Emergency Management Agency (FEMA) trailers had at least one chronic medical condition, compared to a national average of about 13 percent.[4,5]

People who don't live on a sea coast also could find themselves in increased danger of being flooded as inland flood plains expand from more ferocious storms. Consistent with what is expected with a warming climate, heavy rainfall events have become, on average, 24 percent more frequent across the continental United States since 1948, with New England experiencing an increase of more than 60 percent and the Mid-Atlantic states more than a 40 percent increase in flooding.[6]

As an important aside, currently private homeowner's insurance excludes damage from floods. The U.S. government offers flood insurance that homeowners can purchase separately. But it may not be viable for the U.S. government to continue to provide this insurance as the areas at risk of flooding continue to increase, and many people can't afford the additional insurance regardless of who provides it. People who find themselves in a newly designated floodplain could face personal financial ruin if they can't sell their homes or get insurance to protect their investments. Worry about finances is one of the most common causes of mental stress and anxiety, which takes a toll on physical well-being.

## FLOODS, CONTAMINATION, AND DISEASE

Floods also increase our risk for contracting diseases. During an extreme weather event such as Katrina, flooding can contribute to a loss of electrical power and damage to pipelines, buildings, and machinery. Those events, in turn, knock out water and sewage services and compromise residents' ability to maintain good hygiene. Flooding also can bring victims directly into contact with the dirty water that fosters disease.

After Hurricane Katrina, more than a thousand cases of vomiting and diarrhea were reported among evacuees in Houston, Texas. The culprit was determined to be norovirus, a germ often responsible for large outbreaks of diarrhea on cruise ships. Norovirus is particularly easy to pass from person to person as only a tiny amount of the virus can cause disease. Fortunately, if a victim has adequate fluids to prevent dehydration, the body can usually fight off the illness on its own after a few days, and no deaths were reported from norovirus in Houston.[7]

Floods have additional health-harming effects. As floodwaters wash over farms, they pick up manure, chemical fertilizers, and pesticides. As they wash over industrial sites, they also pick up chemicals that have spilled onto the ground or from leaking storage tanks or machinery. And as floodwaters wash over towns and cities, they pick up gas and oil from the streets, garbage, toxins, bacteria and other germs, and everything else that is lying around. All of this floodwater, along with everything it is carrying, then washes into surface waters, such as lakes, rivers, and reservoirs, which supply much of the United States with its drinking water.

Water treatment plants are fairly good at removing normal amounts of bacteria and viruses. When the number of germs in the water increases, however, some germs are not removed or destroyed and end up in our drinking water, explaining why most outbreaks of waterborne disease occur after heavy rains. The most famous outbreak occurred after very heavy rains in Milwaukee, Wisconsin, in 1993. More than 400,000 people became sickened by a germ called cryptosporidium, resulting in 54 deaths.[8] Unfortunately, water treatment plants were not designed to remove chemical toxins, so they can enter our drinking water.

If all this talk of flooding makes you uneasy about where you live, it is reasonable to consider how vulnerable to flooding you might be. If you live in a low-lying coastal area, be aware that the seas will rise. Moving early might allow you to recoup more of your property value. Given the rapidly changing conditions in the Arctic and Antarctic, we can't yet predict with accuracy how much or how fast the waters will rise, but they will rise. It's possible that the sea level will rise enough in the next several decades and combine with hurricanes and storm surges to do substantial damage to coastal property.

Keep in mind, however, that there will be few, if any, places that are completely free from extreme weather events in the era of climate change. Almost every region of the United States has experienced some flooding in its history, and inland floodplains will also expand as a result of more frequent heavy rain events. Tornadoes also routinely plague the heartland and may become more frequent. And although hurricanes— or typhoons—are less common on the West Coast, heavy rains that cause flooding and mudslides, along with droughts, and devastating forest fires that already occur there with disturbing regularity, are expected to become more frequent and more severe with climate change.

Although a place to live that is completely "safe" doesn't exist, it makes sense to examine your vulnerability and try to minimize it as much as possible.

## FLOODS, MOLD, AND MORE

Flooding, hurricanes, and storms also cause moist environments, which can soak walls and floors in housing, creating ideal environments for disease-causing mold to grow. Not only is the mold unsightly, some molds can produce toxins that damage lung tissue when people breathe the air containing them, or they can trigger allergic reactions in sensitive people. The heavier the contamination, the more likely it is that exposed people could suffer illness. Repeated or prolonged exposure probably poses a greater health risk.

Although mold is not always harmful (in fact, penicillin mold is responsible for the first antibiotic ever used!), molds can cause allergic reactions, infections, and even secrete deadly toxins. Individuals who have respiratory conditions, such as asthma or the severe lung disease called chronic obstructive pulmonary disorder (COPD), and persons whose immune systems don't work well, should avoid engaging in activities that would expose them to mold if at all possible. Other groups that might be at higher risk for mold-related illness include pregnant women, senior citizens, and children younger than 12.

The common symptoms of mold exposure, such as persistent stuffy or runny nose, sinus congestion or postnasal drip, or red, itchy eyes, might be fairly mild. Those with asthma might experience a worsening of their regular symptoms, including wheezing, shortness of breath, or cough. It is possible for normal, healthy people to experience similar symptoms. Mold can occasionally cause infections, leading to such symptoms as fevers and fatigue. If you are concerned that you might have been exposed to mold and you are experiencing any of these symptoms, see your health care provider.

Exposure to undisturbed mold, however, is unlikely to result in disease. If someone merely goes into a home following a flood to survey damage but doesn't disturb the scene, even if mold is visibly present in large quantities, that person is unlikely to suffer ill effects. People who are working to rehabilitate homes or buildings, including tearing out damaged and moldy materials, such as wallboards, carpets, or flooring, are at greatest risk. They should consult their physicians first to get instructions about the best kind of protective equipment to use for each situation, and sometimes it's best to hire a professional to fix flooded buildings or homes.

After Hurricane Katrina, about half of all homes in the flooded areas were contaminated with mold, and the Centers for Disease Control estimated that many of those homes were heavily contaminated.[9] Mold growth is likely if a building has been wet for more than 48 hours, extensive mold is visible, or signs of water damage are visible and the building has a musty odor. The mold might be growing inside walls, above ceilings, or under floors and might not be obvious. Mold, once it takes hold in a home or building, is difficult but not impossible to remove. Some mold removal tips are included in the solutions section.[10]

Although flooded buildings provide an ideal setting for mold growth, standing water and damp environments that occur after floods and hurricanes also provide ideal living conditions for dust mites, which can worsen asthma, and bacteria, which can cause allergic reactions and lung infections. Standing water also encourages cockroaches and rodents, and many building materials contain toxic chemicals that can be released with prolonged moisture.

## STORM SURGE

We may experience the repercussions of flooding in another way: storm surge. We know that a small rise in sea level can translate into large amounts of storm surge—those crashing waves associated with major storms along coasts—but figuring how much storm surge to expect from a given rise in sea level is tricky. It depends a lot on the local geography and topography of the land, the direction and speed of the wind, the direction the storm is moving, the vegetation present, and what barriers—natural or manmade—lie underwater offshore. As an example, scientists from the NASA Goddard Institute of Space Studies report that today a Category 3 hurricane on a worst-case track could cause 25 feet (7.6 m) of storm surge at John F. Kennedy International Airport in New York City. With an additional rise in sea level, that storm surge could be considerably higher.[11]

Moving from the Big Apple to the Big Easy, we all saw what happened when Category 3 Katrina made landfall close to New Orleans at current sea levels. How much more damage and harm to our health would be done with an additional rise in sea level of 12 inches or more?

## SALTWATER CONTAMINATION OF WELLS

One of the most damaging implications of sea level rise and resultant flooding is the potential for contaminated freshwater wells and aquifers. In the last chapter, we discussed how important clean, fresh water is to maintaining our health. In many coastal areas around the world, including those in the United States, water wells—and the aquifers that provide the water for those wells—are shallow. This is the case even in some areas where human settlements are located on high bluffs.

As sea levels rise, salt water can flow into freshwater wells and aquifers, contaminating the water and rendering it unfit to drink or to use for crop irrigation. In coastal Georgia, for example, special monitors have been placed in wells to alert water managers to saltwater contamination. And residents of low-lying atolls in the Pacific Ocean are being relocated to islands that are higher in elevation as rising seas contaminate their limited freshwater sources.

## EROSION

Rising seas combined with big storms and surges also contribute to the erosion and loss of coastal land, potentially causing the forced evacuation of homes and businesses, loss of property, financial ruin, and mental stress. Some coastal towns are painfully aware of how much land they're already losing. The famous beaches of South Florida have lost so much beach land that they've been dredging sand for "beach renourishment" from the nearby ocean depths for years. Now, there's no more sand to be found locally, and those in charge of keeping the beaches looking inviting are scrambling to buy sand from distant places. They're also considering more creative solutions, such as turning recycled glass bottles into beach sand—not such an outrageous idea if you consider that glass comes from sand in the first place. As the economy in this area depends largely on tourism dollars, not having a beach for the tourists could mean economic ruin for many South Florida communities.[12] But South Florida is certainly not alone in its problems with erosion. By 2060, one in four houses located within 500 feet of the shoreline in U.S. coastal communities could be lost to erosion, according to a special nationwide study commissioned by the U.S. Federal Emergency Management Agency.[13]

Barriers certainly can be erected to protect specific areas from erosion, rising sea level, and storm surge. These barriers fall into two general categories: soft and hard. A common hard barrier is a sea wall to protect high-cost infrastructure, such as cities, that can't readily be moved. Hard barriers are fairly effective but extremely expensive to build. Another drawback is that erosion is worse at the ends of the barrier than if the barrier weren't there at all. That means that the barrier has to extend well beyond the important infrastructure to provide full protection. Another drawback to hard barriers is that they can fail, as the levees did in New

Orleans, putting large numbers of people and buildings at risk. Once a barrier is built, people tend to feel safer behind the barrier and might not take prudent precautions, such as evacuating when faced with subsequent large storms. In addition, the barrier's required height will depend on what we do in the next few years to stabilize the climate. There is evidence in the geologic record that the last time the Earth was 3.5°F (2°C) to 5.5°F (3°C) warmer—well within the range projected for this century—sea levels were 80 feet (25 m) to 115 feet (30 m) higher than they are today![14]

Soft barriers include beaches and coastal vegetation that absorb some of the storm surge and protect areas behind them. Native coastal vegetation has evolved with various survival strategies that help to hold the beach sand in place. Some scientists have estimated, for example, that if the Louisiana bayou between New Orleans and the Gulf had been intact rather than degraded for decades by human activity, the storm surge from Hurricane Katrina could have been reduced considerably.[15] No one will ever know if that difference could have kept the levees from breaking, but there is reason to believe that it might have done so. In the chapter on ecosystems, we'll explain more about the role of healthy coastal ecosystems in protecting coastal communities from erosion and big storms.

## OTHER EFFECTS OF CATACLYSMIC EVENTS ON HEALTH

The storms and other events that will accompany climate change will have other consequences for our health. Thunderstorms are likely to increase, and if they occur during hay fever season when pollen counts are highest many people with asthma and pollen allergies may suffer more. Epidemics of bad asthma attacks associated with thunderstorms have been documented in a number of countries, including Australia, Italy, and the United Kingdom. Researchers say that pollen grains carried on the air currents of thunderstorms can burst with sudden changes in humidity, releasing even smaller particles into the atmosphere. These tiniest of particles can penetrate deeper into the lungs. If a person breathing in these particles is allergic to the pollen, severe asthma attacks can result, sometimes even in people who previously did not have asthma.[16]

Greater storms portend other ill effects for humanity. Apart from their potentially damaging winds, hurricanes, cyclones, and typhoons can dump copious quantities of rain as they come ashore. Hurricane Katrina, for instance, released as much as 15 inches of rain in a few hours around New Orleans.[17] We've already noted that flooding from that kind of rain, especially in already waterlogged areas, is dangerous to human health, but the dangers can present themselves in more ways than you might think. The next section explains.

## RISK TO INFRASTRUCTURE AND HEALTH

Most of us saw on our TV screens after Hurricane Katrina hit New Orleans that we're not terribly good at evacuating many people—especially those with limited means—before a big storm is expected. But we simply can't evacuate infrastructure. *Infrastructure* refers to the facilities, systems, and services of our society's organizational structure. We rely on these large-scale public systems, such as hospitals and clinics, water and sewage treatment plants, garbage disposal, emergency response systems, roads and transportation, telecommunications, grocery stores, schools, and even legal systems, to maintain our health and well-being. As sea levels rise, more and more of the critical infrastructure that we rely on to keep us healthy will be at risk. This situation may force us to consider where to place our biggest and most prestigious hospitals and medical centers, our water and sewage treatment plants, and our emergency response systems, among other important elements of our public health infrastructure. Often such institutions exist in our largest cities, which are disproportionately located in coastal regions. And that's where almost half of the U.S. population lives—within 50 miles of a coastline.[18]

Before Hurricane Katrina slammed into the Gulf Coast in 2005, New Orleans had seven hospitals. Two years after the storm, only one hospital was fully functional, and two others were partially open.[19] More than 200 physicians did not return after the hurricane. Since then, there's been a steady trickle of physicians, particularly specialists, leaving the area.

Moreover, many patients lost their jobs—and their health insurance— after the storm. This situation is another one of those vicious cycles— physicians won't return until there are patients and medical facilities available, but the patients won't return until there are physicians available. Economists have identified the loss of the health-care infrastructure in New Orleans as a major block to economic revival there.[19]

A telephone survey of more than 1,000 Katrina survivors found that about three out of four suffered from a chronic medical condition before the storm hit. One in five of those survivors was unable to continue medical treatment after the storm. The treatment interruptions were due to such factors as an inability to access physicians or medications, loss of insurance and/or financial problems, and a lack of transportation. The study authors believe their survey actually underestimates these problems.[20]

Meanwhile, some parents living in FEMA trailers in Louisiana reported that their children had required repeated emergency room visits and had been hospitalized for severe asthmatic episodes because they couldn't get their children's asthma medications. Some children who had seen physicians after the storm were not put back on their previous medications because their past medical history could not be checked. Overall, these parents were three times more likely to report that their children's health was fair or poor compared to national averages.[4] The fact that health-care providers couldn't access the medical records of disaster survivors—which electronic medical records might prevent—may have exacerbated the children's problems.[20]

Health may be compromised even more after a disaster if people become poorer as a result. And the already poor suffer the most: One in every two households with an annual income of less than $10,000 before Hurricane Katrina lost all of its salaried jobs after the storm, whereas only one in six households with an annual income of more than $20,000 before the storm lost its jobs thereafter. Moreover, children in coastal Mississippi were twice as likely to be uninsured after Hurricane Katrina, resulting in many children not seeking care for illness or injury.[21]

Some insurance companies appear to understand how critical infrastructure is to society—and how costly it can be to replace or rebuild infrastructure following a weather disaster. Large international re-insurance companies (companies that insure the insurance companies), such as Swiss Re, have been at the forefront of discussions about whether the climate is changing, who is causing it, and what can be done about it. These companies have been quick to point out that weather-related losses recently have resulted in skyrocketing losses for covered damages.[22] Allstate Corporation responded to this in 2006 by announcing that it would no longer offer homeowner's insurance to coastal communities in Maryland. Allstate also has stopped covering homeowners in Delaware, Connecticut, New Jersey, and parts of Virginia. Meanwhile, residents in New York, the Carolinas, and Texas have had trouble renewing their policies. Following substantial losses in Florida and the Gulf Coast during the past few years, several insurance companies have raised their rates precipitously or dropped coverage altogether for businesses and residences in these areas.[23]

## DISPLACED PEOPLE

The rising sea levels, storms, and floods associated with climate change will soon displace millions of people globally. The fleeing of tens of thousands of Gulf Coast residents from Hurricane Katrina could be just a preview of the devastation to come. Some countries, though, could have it much worse than others. Experts at the U.N. Environment Programme have estimated that if the sea level in the Bay of Bengal rises by three feet (1 m), Bangladesh will lose almost a sixth of its land mass. Moreover, the land at risk of flooding is where much of the country's rice production occurs. This is a double whammy for Bangladesh, an already crowded country with more than 150 million people (half the population of the United States) living in an area about the size of North Carolina. As millions of people are displaced from their homes and farms there, they face the challenge of finding space in a crowded country, and their ability to feed themselves will also be severely compromised by the loss of land for rice production.

Bangladesh is almost completely surrounded by India, another very crowded country. If displaced Bangladesh residents try to move into India, which is already struggling to feed its own people, additional conflict could result. In fact, the World Bank has identified 10 "poor countries" that will be at especially high risk due to a rise in sea level. In addition to Bangladesh, Benin, Guyana, Surinam, Guinea-Bissau, Egypt, Mauritania, Gambia, Vietnam, and Sri Lanka are all at high risk from a rise in sea level.[24]

Civilization largely developed along the coasts of land masses because of the availability of sea travel. As a result, 13 of the 20 largest cities in the world are located at sea level. A three-foot (1-m) rise in sea level is likely to displace hundreds of millions of people during this century.[24] The forced migration of these people combined with already scarce resources in many of these areas—and municipal and national infrastructures that are stressed by current populations—is a recipe for disaster and could lead to escalating conflict.

## CONFLICT

Of course, conflict is bad for our health. In addition to people being killed and injured during conflict, social systems are disrupted, increasing the risk of illness or death from other threats, such as famine and infectious disease.[25] Furthermore, the relative wealth of the United States and the ever-widening gap between the haves and the have-nots will continue to draw both legal and illegal immigrants to the United States and to other industrialized nations as they seek the means to provide shelter and food for their families in a resource-constricted world. Real and perceived competition for scarce resources here in the United States may escalate tensions between races, ethnicities, religions, and those of differing immigration status.

## CATACLYSMIC EVENTS AND MENTAL HEALTH

The experience of displacement and conflict from rising seas, surging waters, floods, and other destruction associated with climate change will be an enormous blow to the mental well-being of millions of Earth's citizens.[26] Hurricane Katrina showed us that storms coupled with a rise in sea level and inadequate flood management can result in devastating alterations to the victims' way of life, upending both their physical and psychological balance.

Although many people only have normal, short-term reactions of stress, grief, anger, sadness, anxiety, guilt, and poor sleep, extreme disaster experiences can lead to long-term post-traumatic stress—an illness that occurs when victims relive their traumatic experiences over and over in their minds, avoid anything that reminds them of the trauma they experienced, and remain persistently aroused or anxious.[27-29] Other forms of anxiety, depression, family problems, difficulties at work, child misbehavior, poor academic functioning, a sense of lost identity, and a host of other symptoms also may occur as a result of these experiences.[30-32] Moreover, people who have anxiety and depression before these climatic disasters are more likely to experience severe reactions in response to them.[33,34]

The research on mental suffering after floods and other natural disasters is sobering. After Hurricane Katrina, one study showed that mental illness doubled.[35] One year after Hurricane Katrina, children of affected families were four times more likely than before the storm to have a diagnosis of depression or anxiety and twice as likely to have behavioral problems.[21] Although these psychological problems often diminish, they also can persist or be rekindled at the anniversary of the initial disaster.[1,31]

Other studies on how adults and children respond to such climatic disasters as tornadoes also indicate they are at higher risk for long-term, severe mental health problems, including anxiety, post-traumatic stress, and depression.[36-38]

Many people also have mental health disabilities related to physical injury, disease, malnutrition, and lack of access to clean water, which often occur in the aftermath of disasters.[39] And, of course, when people are forced out of their homes and communities to move to already stressed places and compete with the local people for scarce resources, an increased risk of poor mental health outcomes can arise.[26]

For many people, global warming also will produce so much climatic variability—say, severe storms followed by droughts—that they will find it difficult to cope with the unpredictability.[40] The stresses of climate change are more likely to affect persons with fewer financial resources or members of minority populations who may sense less community support.[1] Regardless of a person's socioeconomic situation, a sense of security in daily routine may be threatened in the face of climate change.

One final mental health note is needed here. We often justify the misery that victims of natural disasters experience by blaming them for their plight or by accepting the unjust dynamics, such as poverty and lack of access to resources, that make them more likely to be victimized.[41] If we simply accept the status quo or blame the victims, it may compound the psychological suffering of millions of people dealing with climate change's harm around the world in years to come.

## THE SCIENCE OF A RISE IN SEA LEVEL

Now that you have a better idea of how the cataclysmic events induced by climate change may harm us, it's instructive to understand some of the science underlying two of the more complicated events. Let's begin with a rise in sea level.

### Thermal Expansion

The sea level is already slightly higher than it was a century ago. As neither Greenland nor Antarctica have melted much yet, why is the sea higher? The main reason is because of thermal expansion. Heat makes things expand. Warm water takes up more space than cold water. And because the oceans are contained by more or less stationary continental land masses, the main direction their waters have for expansion is up as Earth's temperature rises.

### Melting Inland Glaciers

Although melting ice has not yet contributed as much as thermal expansion to rising sea levels, it will. The inland glaciers of North America, the Swiss Alps, the Himalayas, and the South American Andes are melting quickly.[42] As these glaciers melt, the fresh water drains into rivers and eventually into the sea. Most inland glaciers will be largely melted by 2100, leaving one-sixth of the world's population without its main water source.[43] The Andean glaciers of South America are expected to melt even more rapidly and be gone in a few decades.[44] Although these inland glaciers provide vast amounts of fresh water for more than 1 billion people, their contribution to global sea-level rise will be relatively minuscule, between four and ten inches (0.1 to 0.25 m).[45]

## Greenland's Melting Ice

By comparison, Greenland, a vast ice sheet of glaciers about three times the size of Texas and almost two miles (3 km) thick, will add an estimated 21 feet (6.4 meters) to global sea levels when it melts completely.[42] And it may be melting faster than anticipated. Huge holes have formed in the surface of Greenland's glaciers, some as much as 45 feet (15 m) across and with meltwater pouring into the holes.[46] That water, which always seeks the easiest path and is constantly being pulled down by gravity, is traversing these holes to the bottom of the glaciers. It then flows between the bottom of the glaciers and the bedrock, effectively "greasing the skids" of the glaciers and speeding their movement to the sea. Greenland's glaciers had been poking along but are now moving about 10 miles (15 km) per year with periodic lurches. One amazing surge was measured at three miles (5 km) in just 90 minutes. This type of new glacier activity is why scientists now believe Greenland is melting far faster than they had expected.

And although the global average temperature increase during the past century was just 1°F (0.5°C), the temperature on the Greenland ice sheet has increased by 7°F (3.9°C) just since 1991.[47] This greater warming over the ice has not only led to the extended summer surface melt on Greenland but also to the loss of summer sea ice in the Arctic.

## Melting Arctic Sea Ice

Every summer, some of the ice in the Arctic Sea around the North Pole melts, usually reaching its lowest point sometime in mid-September before expanding again during the winter. During the past six years, more and more of the sea ice has melted away during the summer whereas the winter expansions have been less vigorous. (Melting sea ice doesn't contribute to rising sea levels because it's already floating in the sea, but as we'll see in a moment it creates other climate change problems.)

Up until the summer of 2007, the Arctic Sea always had ice blocking the passage of ships *somewhere* all year round—ever since humans began building ships. The Arctic Sea hit its lowest summer ice mass ever during the week of September 16, 2007.[47] At that time, ships had clear passage for the first time. Some nations and businesses are looking at this event with enthusiasm, envisioning quicker oceanic transportation times between the East and West.

But the loss of Arctic Sea ice means more to the world than the faster transport of goods. (See Figure 6.1.) Ice is very good at *reflecting* much of the Sun's energy—80 percent, to be exact—back out into space. When the ice melts it leaves dark sea water exposed, which *absorbs* 90 percent of the Sun's energy and further warms the planet, which melts more ice and causes more warming.[48] Hence, the melting sea ice leads to another one of those dangerous feedback loops and could lead to much warmer temperatures occurring far more rapidly than originally thought.

The summer of 2007 saw more than 1 million square miles (2.6 million square km) of dark Arctic Sea water exposed beyond the average since 1979, when satellites began making such measurements possible.[49] Scientists have long been concerned about the possibility of *abrupt* climate change. This refers to the idea that the Earth may not warm up gradually but instead experience events that would trigger abrupt increases in warming. Time and further studies are needed to know if the extreme Arctic Sea ice melt during the summer of 2007 was just a freak occurrence or the start of an ominous trend. And the positive feedback loops discussed in this book are the most likely mechanisms for abrupt climate change to occur.

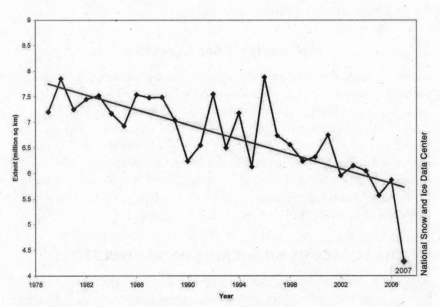

**Figure 6.1**   Graph showing rapid decline of Arctic Sea ice since 1978.

## Melting Antarctica

Antarctica in the Southern Hemisphere, in contrast to the Arctic, is mostly composed of ice that is not floating. Antarctica connects with land underwater, so as its ice melts it does contribute to a rise in sea level. Although some parts of the colder, drier interior of Antarctica are still expected to gain ice from increased snowfall, the continent has experienced a net loss of ice mass and has already melted more rapidly than scientists thought possible.[50] Some parts of Antarctica are massive ice sheets extending over the water, and two of these sheets have already collapsed. "Larsen A" collapsed in 1995, and the Rhode Island-sized "Larsen B" collapsed quite suddenly in 2002. Those ice sheets didn't add much to sea-level rise, but they were behaving like dams, holding the large glaciers behind them in place. Now that the dams have been removed, the glaciers can flow more quickly to the sea.

The Texas-sized West Antarctic Ice Sheet, located south of South America, has its base deep under the surface of the Southern Ocean and can be seen as sitting on pillars of ice in the water. As the Southern Ocean warms up, these pillars of ice are melting, threatening to break the entire ice sheet off into the water. If this happens, global sea levels will increase by 15 to 21 feet (4.6 to 6.4 m).[51] And if Antarctica melts completely, it would contribute another 200 feet to sea-level rise, although scientists don't expect that to happen soon and are more worried about the melting of the West Antarctic Ice Sheet.

## Melting Ice = Sea-Level Rise

Taken together, the polar caps and our glaciers are melting faster than scientists predicted even a few years ago. As a result, sea levels will rise during this century by at least a couple of feet and maybe six feet (2 m) or more.[14] Even modest amounts of sea-level rise will have grave implications for the health and well-being of people all over the world, including those in the United States, by inundating or completely submerging homes, communities, and cropland; causing injury and death from higher storm surge and flooding; contaminating freshwater supplies; and adding to societal instability and threats to global security.

## THE SCIENCE OF HURRICANES AND OTHER STORMS

Atlantic hurricanes—the ones we experience the most in the United States—can work in concert with sea-level rise to do much of their damage. Hurricanes typically start over the warm tropical waters off the west coast of Africa. When the water's surface temperature is at least 80°F (26.7°C), evaporation from the ocean's surface creates higher humidity in the atmosphere, which then spawns thunderstorms. When the powerful thunderstorms converge and begin to rotate in the atmosphere, this whirling mass of air and moisture, called a tropical depression, draws heat from the ocean's surface up through its center resulting in high winds and rain around the outside of the depression. The warmer the surface water, the more energy is available to produce heavy rains and high winds, which explains why global warming may contribute to stronger hurricanes.

Once a depression's wind speeds top 35 miles per hour (56 km/h), the system officially becomes a tropical storm and the National Hurricane Center gives it a name. If the storm intensifies to sustained wind speeds of 74 miles per hour (119 km/h), it becomes a Category 1 hurricane. Hurricanes are divided into five categories based on their wind speeds. A Category 5 hurricane, currently the strongest category, must have sustained wind speeds greater than 155 miles per hour (250 km/h). Although Hurricane Katrina reached Category 5 status over the Gulf of Mexico, she had weakened to a Category 3 by the time she hit the Louisiana-Mississippi coast with winds of about 125 miles per hour (201 km/h). The hurricane's winds whip up the ocean's surface, causing waves, or a storm surge, from 4 to 5 feet (1.2 to 1.5 m) for a Category 1 hurricane to more than 18 feet (5.5 m) for a Category 5 hurricane.[52]

In addition to the surface temperature of the sea, plenty of other factors are involved in determining the formation and strength of a hurricane, including wind patterns and other regional and global weather events. You've likely heard of El Niño, which occurs when the waters of the Pacific Ocean close to the equator warm up and create different global wind patterns that tend to cause more typhoons in the Pacific but fewer hurricanes in the Atlantic. Often, during the year after El Niño comes La Niña, which produces cooler ocean temperatures in the Pacific Ocean leading to more frequent and severe Atlantic hurricanes.

Although hurricane researchers have not reached consensus, there is increasing evidence that warmer ocean temperatures from climate change contribute to stronger and perhaps more frequent hurricanes.[53-55] Some researchers have documented an increasing number of Category 4 and 5 storms in the past 35 years.[56,57] The connection between warmer ocean temperatures and hurricanes is especially strong in the Atlantic Ocean, but other factors may be stronger in the Pacific Ocean.[58] The complexity of hurricane formation makes accurate projections more difficult. Further research is needed to better under-stand how hurricane strength and frequency will be affected by climate change.

Small-scale extreme weather events such as tornadoes and hailstorms occur locally and sporadically, making it difficult to gather sufficient data to determine long-term trends related to climate change. Recent research, however, suggests that the cooling rain that occurs as hurricanes weaken when they make landfall could make the formation of tornadoes more likely.[59] And there is no question that climate change will bring more extreme weather events, including episodes of heavy rainfall and thunderstorms.

## SOLUTIONS

### Individual Solutions

- Do everything possible to reduce your greenhouse gas emissions and stabi-lize the climate quickly to help reduce cataclysmic weather events.
- Take precautions to protect yourself and your family from these events, because some are inevitable. Begin with a family emergency plan and an emergency preparedness kit. (Additional information about emergency plans and kits can be found at www.ready.gov.)
  - Have a personal and family emergency communication plan.
  - Know several routes to get to hospitals and out of town.
  - Have a personal and family emergency evacuation plan for all places in which you and your family spend a lot of time, including, home, work, and school.
  - In the event of an emergency, listen to your television or radio and follow the advice and instructions the authorities give.
  - If the authorities recommend evacuation—evacuate! Gather up your emergency preparedness kit, family, pets, relatives, and neighbors, and move to a safer place.
  - As silly as it may sound, practice your emergency plans with your entire family regularly.
  - Assemble an emergency preparedness kit—see box on page 97 for a list of suggested contents. Consider having an emergency preparedness kit at home, in the car, and at work.
  - Purchase flood insurance. Special flood insurance must be purchased from the U.S. government. Information can be found at http://www.fema.gov/business/nfip/.

## Emergency Preparedness Kit

Your personal or family emergency preparedness kit should contain at minimum the following items:

- One gallon of water for *each person* (and each sizeable pet) *per day* for at least a three-day supply
- Nonperishable food, preferably food that doesn't need to be cooked, for at least three days
- Can opener
- First-aid kit
- Bottle of hand sanitizer and moist towelettes
- At least a three-day supply of any medications needed
- AM radio, preferably one that can be recharged with a hand crank
- Flashlights, preferably ones that can be recharged with a hand crank
- Extra batteries
- Cash (if there's no electricity, a credit card is just a piece of plastic)
- Identification
- Warm clothing, emergency blankets, rain gear
- Baby or children's items, if appropriate
- Whistle
- Medical equipment or supplies, such as oxygen, if required for survival or well-being, with spares if possible
- A list of everything that should be in the kit
- Check your kit for completeness, make sure everything works, and replace food, water, medicines, and batteries annually. Even water in unopened plastic bottles should be replaced regularly.

## Mold Removal

Mold removal and cleanup should be performed by a professional if possible, especially if a lot of mold is present. If this isn't possible or there is only a small amount of mold, follow these instructions:[10]

- Wear rubber boots, rubber gloves, and goggles.
- Open windows and doors to allow as much fresh air to come in as possible.
- Set up dehumidifiers and fans pointing outward toward open doors and windows to remove moisture from the area.
- Items that are porous and have soaked up water but can't be put into a washing machine or dry-cleaned should be removed and discarded.

- Nonporous surfaces should be scrubbed (gloves on!) with a solution of one cup of bleach mixed with one gallon of water. Rinse the item with clean water and allow it to dry thoroughly.
- Never mix bleach-containing products with products containing ammonia—the resulting fumes can be fatal!

## Community Solutions

- Communities require their own disaster preparedness plans, including resources for evacuation and shelters for citizens to make sure they are safe and have access to vital resources if needed.
- Communities also need to help citizens, especially the poor and underserved, become physically and mentally prepared for disasters to reduce potential harmful health and mental health outcomes.
- Communities should focus on improving social support and connecting people with resources to help foster their resiliency so they will be able to cope in the aftermath of disasters.
- Citizens can get involved in the following zoning issues, which are usually decided locally and allow citizen input:
  - Consider the potential harm from rising sea levels and/or expanding floodplains in your area. Seek outside experts to help with this assessment.
  - Stop building in these high-risk areas.
  - Consider voluntary relocation programs for people already living in high-risk areas.
  - Use community funds for these efforts. This is a good investment, considering the high social and economic costs of major damage and rebuilding.

## Regional, National, and International Solutions

- Encourage state and national governments to provide incentives for voluntary relocation programs for people already living in high-risk areas.
- Protect and reconstruct coastal and wetland ecosystems to minimize storm damage farther inland.
- Wetlands are instrumental in controlling flooding. Consider allowing inland flood plains to return to or become natural wetland preserves.

# Chapter 7

## Infectious Disease: Bacteria, Viruses, and Parasites, Oh My

Maria doesn't know what to think about Arnie's call. He sounds worried, but he also sounds resigned as he describes his symptoms: high fever, a blistering headache, deep, throbbing pains in his joints, and muscle fatigue.

"Arnie, you've likely just got the flu," Maria tells her brother on the crackling cell phone call. "All of your symptoms point to the flu."

"How can this be the flu when it's not even cold yet?" was his weary reply. "I feel terrible in this darned heat. And what about this rash?"

"What rash?" Maria asks. "This is the first time you've mentioned a rash. Have you gone to see your doctor?"

"Nah, he's too busy," Arnie says. "He can't see me until next week."

"So what's this rash?" she asks again.

Maria hasn't talked to Arnie since she learned two days ago that Max is bringing his entire family to live with her and her family because of the approaching hurricane and possible final destruction to his home. She doesn't know what to say to Arnie, especially because she feels guilty about doubting his ability to handle anything too stressful.

"It's not so bad," Arnie replies, describing the redness on his knees and thighs. "I mean, it's red and warm and all that. Everything else hurts much more."

Maria mulls over his symptoms—a rash plus fever, headaches, and deep pain in his joints and muscles. It couldn't be, Maria thinks to herself, allowing a silence in the conversation that unnerves Arnie.

"So what are you thinking, M?" Arnie asks, stress in his voice.

"Well, have you ever heard of dengue fever?"

"I think so," he says, uneasy. "On the news recently, maybe."

"It's been in the southern parts of the United States," Maria says, "but this climate change has been helping it move northward. The mosquitoes that carry it like the new warmth up north. I don't recall hearing of any cases in New York, but . . ."

"But what?" Arnie asks, sounding more worried now.

"But . . . have you been taking any aspirin for the aches and pains?" she asks, a nervous edge in her voice.

"No, but I was going to take something soon because I'm getting worse."

"Okay, good," Maria hears herself saying almost automatically. "Don't take anything yet. Just get yourself to the emergency room pronto. If it's dengue, it probably won't kill you, but go—now."

Maria listens as Arnie expresses his doubts, shaking her head and wondering what other trouble global warming will bring her family in the coming days, weeks, and months.

## THE RELATIONSHIP BETWEEN CLIMATE AND INFECTIOUS DISEASE

Throughout time humans have suffered from infectious diseases, and climate change will give the parasites, bacteria, and viruses that cause them some new advantages. These germs are sensitive to the temperature of their surroundings, and generally they reproduce and mature more quickly into disease-causing entities in warmer temperatures.

In addition, insects often are the carriers for these germs, and because insects have no internal mechanisms for regulating their body temperatures they benefit from warmer environments. Insects generally hatch earlier and develop more quickly into adults at higher temperatures, and the adults then move from one host to another, taking a blood meal from each. If the insect is infected with a disease, the germs that spread that disease are passed from one "victim" to the next with the insect's bite, causing the infection to spread.

## MALARIA AND CLIMATE CHANGE

Malaria is one of the diseases that climate change already is influencing. In Africa, where it is prevalent, malaria is currently limited by elevation because it must be at least 59°F (15°C) for the malaria parasite to develop inside the mosquito host. The temperature falls, on average, about 11°F (6°C) for every 3,300 feet (1,000 m) gained in elevation. Historically, malaria has rarely occurred above about 3,300 feet (1,000 m) elevation because it was too cold for the disease-causing parasites to develop inside the mosquitoes.[1] As the climate is warming, however, malaria is creeping up into the highlands and infecting populations that have no previous experience with the disease and therefore no protecting immunity. In these populations, malaria is even more devastating than in the populations where it is common. The increases in malaria, however, are not completely out of our control. In the Peruvian Amazon, it was found that deforestation leads to higher malaria rates because the changes in landscape encourage the mosquitoes that carry malaria to thrive, demonstrating again that decisions we make about how we interact with our environment can influence our health.[2]

Could malaria become a problem in the United States? Believe it or not, malaria once *was* a problem here. Before World War II, malaria was a common problem in the southeastern United States. It didn't cease being a problem because it got colder there. The Centers for Disease Control and Prevention are located in Atlanta, Georgia, because the agency was initially created from a branch of the Public Health Service called the Malaria Control in War Areas, which was charged with keeping the many military bases in the southeastern states malaria-free during World War II. As research uncovered ways to control the spread of malaria, primarily by the use of insecticides such as DDT, the war against malaria was gradually won, and the United States was declared malaria free in 1949.

Clearly temperature is not the only important factor involved in whether a disease like malaria can take hold and become a problem. To this day, about 1,200 cases of malaria are discovered in the United States every year.[3] Most malaria is brought in by people who contract the disease in other parts of the world and return home with the parasites already inside them. When that occurs, medical institutions make the diagnosis and prescribe the appropriate drugs, and the infected patients are closely monitored to make sure the treatment is completely effective. In addition, public health agencies conduct tests to determine if mosquitoes located in the vicinity of the infected people are themselves infected with the malaria parasites. If they are, insecticides are used to get rid of the infected mosquitoes, preventing the disease from spreading further. As temperatures get warmer, the area suitable for malaria transmission here in the United States will certainly get larger, and the number of people at risk of getting malaria could grow as well—but a large resurgence of malaria is not very likely. In essence, the local medical and public health infrastructure keeps the disease at bay here now, and if we continue to maintain these systems we shouldn't need to worry much about malaria becoming an epidemic here in the future. As malaria increases globally in response to global warming, however, it will be increasingly important that our public health systems work well and are properly funded.

## OTHER DISEASES MOSQUITOES CARRY

Temperature is one environmental feature critical to the development of insects and disease, but others are important as well. Many insects need a certain amount of humidity in the air to survive. And mosquitoes, for example, must have water available to lay their eggs. The eggs hatch into larvae, which swim around in the water and eat decaying plant matter until they mature into the familiar winged adult form we know so well. During droughts, there may be less water around to provide egg-laying habitat, but the other aspects of droughts can actually make the spread of some diseases, including those carried by mosquitoes, more of a problem. When there are droughts, for example, people may store water in containers for longer periods of time. Those storage containers can make great breeding grounds for some insects, notably the mosquitoes that carry dengue fever.

Dengue fever, also known as "breakbone fever" because of how it makes you feel when you get it, has been on the rise globally since about 1950. In South and Central America, the disease has been increasing dramatically since the early 1980s and has been steadily moving northward into the Caribbean and Texas. The Asian tiger mosquito (*Aedes albopictus*) came to the United States in 1985 and has since spread to 36 states. This mosquito is not the primary carrier of dengue fever in parts of the world where dengue epidemics are currently occurring, but it is an acceptable secondary carrier. You may have seen these mosquitoes in your own neighborhoods. Their black- and white-striped legs and body are quite recognizable, and the mosquitoes have gained notoriety as being voracious biters during the daytime. As the dengue virus moves northward, some health officials, including Dr. Anthony Fauci, head of the National Institute of Allergy and Infectious Diseases, worry that dengue fever could become a problem in the United States, transmitted by the Asian tiger mosquitoes that already live in many of the states or by the primary carrier mosquito (*Aedes aegypti*) as it expands its range northward.

Although dengue fever does make people very ill, most recover. There is a less common form of the disease called dengue hemorrhagic fever, however, which causes the victim to bleed internally and is often fatal. The World Health Organization reports that about 22,000 people, mostly children, die from this disease every year.[4] In 1990, about one-third of the world's population was at risk of contracting dengue fever. Computer modeling suggests that by 2050, climate change could put as many as 50 to 60 percent of the global population at risk.[5]

It may be that global warming's influence on climate variability, more than simply its influence on warming temperatures, may be a leading contributor to outbreaks of insect-borne diseases, according to Dr. Paul Epstein, one of the leading experts on the effects of climate change on infectious diseases.[6] As described in the chapter on water, West Nile virus is an example of such a disease. The combination of warmer winters and hot, dry summers provided the ideal conditions for this disease to take hold and spread quickly in the United States once the virus had arrived from distant shores as a side effect of globalization. West Nile virus causes *encephalitis*, an infection of the brain. As of November 2007, more than 27,000 Americans have contracted this disease, although fewer than 1,100 have died from it.[7] The elderly are especially vulnerable to West Nile virus.

Other mosquito-carried viruses that can cause similar infections in the United States are Western equine encephalitis and Eastern equine encephalitis, which generally cause fewer than five cases per year but can be fatal, and La Crosse and St. Louis encephalitis, which usually cause several hundred Americans to become ill every year.[3] St. Louis encephalitis, in particular, may become more of a problem in the future. This virus requires a temperature of 63°F (17°C) to develop inside the mosquito. Researchers discovered that increasing the temperature by even a few degrees significantly increased the transmission season in California, causing it to overlap into the autumn when many older Americans arrive from elsewhere to spend the winter.[8]

## DISEASES FROM OTHER INSECTS

Climate change will affect other insect-borne diseases too. Fleas transmit plague from rodents to people. Plague can still be found in several areas of the world, including the desert Southwest of the United States where people occasionally contract the disease after coming in contact with an infected rodent. Thanks to antibiotics and better watchfulness, plague is no longer the Black Death terror that it was in the Middle Ages—when the disease wiped out more than 25 percent of Europe's population in about one year in the middle of the fourteenth century. Nevertheless, it can still cause serious disease. Recently, a team of researchers working in Kazakhstan, another area of the world where plague is found in rodents, discovered that an increase of just 1.8°F (1°C) in the average springtime temperature led to a 50 percent increase in the number of infected rodents.[9] In New Mexico, researchers found that there were more human plague cases following wetter winter-spring periods. The reason for the increase appears to be that the increased rain leads to more food availability, which increases the rodent population. Also, higher humidity may help fleas survive longer.[10] The more infected rodents there are, the greater the chance that humans will come into contact with one and get plague. Climate change is expected to raise temperatures, and more of the annual rainfall is expected to fall in the winter months, potentially leading to a resurgence of this disease. We will require a strong public health system to detect the increase and control it.

Another illness insects carry is Lyme disease, which has received a lot of media exposure in the United States and is a big concern in the Northeast, Mid-Atlantic, and upper Midwest. Lyme disease is carried by ticks, specifically the "deer tick" (*Ixodes scapularis*). Deer ticks are smaller than dog ticks and are found primarily in wooded areas, rather than in homes and backyards. Ticks, like other insects, are susceptible to changes in climate, and researchers in Sweden have discovered that Lyme disease and other diseases ticks carry are being reported farther and farther north. On the other hand, some of the southern parts of Europe are becoming too warm to support large tick populations.[11] Climate change may be contributing to a rise in tick-borne diseases, mostly because the resulting milder winters and the early arrival of spring prolongs the season during which tick-human encounters can occur.

An additional reason for the increase in cases of Lyme disease in the United States may be the way we are using our land resources. As suburbs expand into surrounding fields and forests and more of the population moves into these areas— behavior that contributes to climate change!— there are more opportunities for humans to come into contact with deer ticks. Another part of the explanation is more complex and involves the health of forest ecosystems and the loss of biodiversity, which we'll explain in the chapter on ecosystems.

Another jump in human disease occurred in 1993 in the Four Corners area of the U.S. Southwest when previously healthy young adults suddenly fell victim to a severe form of pneumonia and died. After some excellent medical sleuthing, the infecting culprit was identified as hantavirus, a previously unknown agent of disease in North America that deer mice carry. Victims were exposed to the virus when they came into contact with airborne particles of dried mouse urine or feces. More than half of those who became ill died. Researchers then learned that the unusually heavy rains in 1991 and 1992 and the extremely mild winter of

1992 had created favorable environmental conditions for an explosion of the deer mouse population.[12] El Niño was blamed for that particular situation, but the combination of environmental events seen during El Niño also describes the conditions that are likely to occur with climate change. During the spring of 2007, Russia reported thousands of cases of hantavirus infections, attributed to an unusually warm winter resulting in a population explosion among the rodents that carry the virus. We may see much more of this disease as climate change brings warmer temperatures and changes in rainfall patterns.

## DISEASES CARRIED ON OCEAN AND WIND CURRENTS

Infectious diseases can be transported around the world in a number of ways. The most common route is when an infected person travels to a new region and spreads the disease upon arrival at his destination. In this way, colonialism contributed to the deaths of tens of thousands of native peoples in South and Central America when the Spanish conquistadors introduced smallpox and measles to the locals who had never been exposed to them before.[13] With globalization, we've certainly seen a lot of this type of spread. Sexually transmitted diseases, the most devastating being HIV/AIDS, are spread effectively in this way. Unsuspecting travelers carried SARS (Sudden Acute Respiratory Syndrome), which started in China, to about 30 countries, including the United States and Canada. This viral infection sickened more than 8,000 people and caused at least 774 deaths before health officials were able to get the disease under control.[14]

Other agents of disease can travel with air and water currents. Cholera, a severely debilitating and often fatal disease, has been shown to hitch a ride with tiny insect-like water creatures called copepods, which look sort of like tiny shrimp and are barely visible without a microscope. The copepods float along on the sea surface on existing ocean currents to new coastal locations where tidal waters carry them—and their cholera-causing bacteria—into rivers and estuaries. Warmer sea surface temperatures encourage blooms of the algae that feed the copepods, resulting in a population explosion of these carriers. Once cholera bacteria are present in the water, people get the disease by ingesting contaminated water or food.[15] So, with warmer temperatures we may see more frequent outbreaks of cholera.

A distant relative of cholera causes trouble for people who love to eat oysters. During the summer of 2004, passengers aboard a cruise ship in Alaska became ill with food poisoning. It was soon discovered that they had been infected when they ate locally harvested fresh oysters. The infectious agent (*Vibrio parahaemolyticus*) had previously only infected oysters in warmer waters. Since 1997, the Alaskan waters where the oysters were harvested had grown warmer by one-fifth of a degree Fahrenheit every year. Eventually, in 2004, the water temperature became warm enough for the virus to grow and flourish, extending its known range by more than 600 miles.[16]

In the chapter about air quality, we discussed dust that carried mold spores from Africa to the Caribbean and Florida. However, the dust that carries these spores doesn't have to come from Africa. A fungus (*Coccidioides immitis*, sometimes called "Cocci" for short) that lives in the U.S. Southwest desert causes an illness called valley fever. When the soil in these areas is disturbed, valley fever spores are thrown into the air. People who have lived all their lives in the region where valley fever is common usually breathe in the spores when they are young, and often they don't get very sick before developing immunity to further infection. When people from other parts of the country or world arrive in the Southwest, however, they have no immunity to the disease and can get a very serious lung infection.

This is a major problem for the thousands of older Americans who have retired to the sunny Southwest from elsewhere. According to the Arizona Department of Health Services, more than 5,500 cases of valley fever were reported in Arizona in 2006, with the vast majority occurring in people older than 65. The average length of the illness was about two months, and 40 percent of its victims were hospitalized, resulting in 33 deaths.[17] At the Pleasant Valley State Prison in central California, more than 900 inmates and 80 prison employees have become ill with valley fever, resulting in more than a dozen inmate deaths in the past three years. New construction stirring up the soil has been blamed for the surge in new cases, but experts are uncertain if other factors have been involved. Valley fever is more of a problem during drought conditions that have been preceded by flooding—conditions that are expected to become more common with climate change.[15]

## FOODBORNE DISEASES

Because disease-causing agents grow and replicate faster in warmer temperatures, food poisoning is expected to increase with global warming. The time that food can safely remain unrefrigerated will decrease with increasing temperatures. Researchers have shown that as the temperature increases, the number of salmonella food poisoning cases will increase as well.[18]

English and Welsh researchers looking at another common cause of food poisoning, a bacteria called Campylobacter, found that an increasing number of cases of this ailment occurred from 1990 to 1999. Ambient temperature seemed to be the most important indicator of that increase. They also found that children under the age of five suffered most often from food poisoning, and boys got sick more often than girls. The researchers cautioned, however, that because they were only looking at cases of food poisoning reported to physicians, their results might have been biased toward children falling ill. Adults might be more willing to "sick it out" at home and not feel the need to see their doctors.[19]

## WHAT'S NEXT?

The most frightening infectious disease that could be made worse from a changing climate is the one we don't know about yet. Emerging infectious diseases are very real concerns; they often infect a lot of people and do a lot of damage before health experts can figure out what's causing each disease and work out a solution to stop it. Climate change may give some diseases an advantage, increasing the number of victims and human suffering. As is the case with many threats to our health, the most vulnerable members of our societies—our children and the elderly, as well as those with the fewest resources—will be hit hardest. Maintaining a strong public health system and stabilizing the climate as quickly as possible will help to reduce the number of people suffering from infectious diseases.

## INFECTIOUS DISEASE AND MENTAL HEALTH

Infectious disease outbreaks that have their roots in climate change are likely to engender a host of mental health problems. While there is no research yet on the interconnections among infectious diseases, global warming, and psychological responses, the studies on the SARS epidemic may be illustrative. They indicate that people responded with enormous anxiety, including post-traumatic stress and depression, to the threats SARS posed.[20–22] Some of those reactions, moreover, were persistent long after the epidemic abated.

Other research indicates that an outbreak of infectious disease can induce a delayed reaction of intense anxiety in children, especially when the children were already anxious to begin with.[23]

Many of the diseases themselves cause mental symptoms too. Malaria, for example, can severely affect a child's ability to think and do well academically, and it can harm speech and language skills and a child's ability to pay attention.[24–27] Dengue fever can induce mental confusion and changes in consciousness in children.[28] West Nile virus also causes a variety of mental symptoms, including problems with concentration, memory, and decision making that last months after the initial infection for 20 percent or more of those sickened.[29]

Importantly, few of our institutions are prepared to deal with the mental health implications of infectious disease or other disasters related to climate change. One study surveyed nongovernmental organizations that intervene after disease epidemics and other disasters and found that fewer than half of them even addressed mental health issues. Of those that did, few of them launched emergency mental health programs in response to crises.[30]

## SOLUTIONS

### Individual Solutions

To reduce your risk of getting an infectious disease carried by an insect:

- Cover up. The best way to avoid catching a disease carried by insects is to avoid getting bitten. If possible, wear long sleeves, long pants, shoes and socks, and a hat when you are outside.
- Avoid being outside during peak insect activity for the disease-carrying insect of concern.
- If you must be outside and have exposed skin, use insect repellent. The U.S. Environmental Protection Agency suggests either DEET or Picaridin as active ingredients. DEET is safe to use on children older than two months of age. Put the repellent on your hands first and then rub it on the child. Do not put repellent on a small child's hands because they'll likely put them in their mouths eventually. [31]
- It is okay to use sunscreen while using DEET repellents, but do not use products that combine sunscreen with DEET. Sunscreens generally need to be reapplied throughout the day. DEET should only be applied once a day.
- When you return indoors, wash all treated skin with soap and water.
- Permethrin is approved for use as an insecticide and repellent on clothing and bed nets only. Follow instructions on the product label carefully.
- Before traveling to another country, check the Centers for Disease Control (CDC) Travelers' Health Web site for specific instructions on how to avoid the diseases that are a problem at your destination.

- If use of any repellent product causes irritation or any other reaction, discontinue use and contact your health care provider.
- For more information, check the CDC Web site.[32]

To reduce your risk of getting other infectious diseases:

- Wash your hands regularly with soap and water, especially after using the bathroom and before eating. The rubbing action of the hand-washing process does the most good.
- Do not use soap that contains antibiotics. There is no evidence that it gets your hands any cleaner, and there is good evidence that when the antibiotics get washed into the sewer and are discharged into surface waters the antibiotic persists. This encourages bacteria to become resistant to antibiotics, reducing the effectiveness of these drugs when you really need them.
- Ask your health care providers, including nurses and medical technicians, to wash their hands or change their gloves before touching you.
- Wash food well, especially food that won't be cooked, before eating it.
- Boil suspect water.
- Avoid eating local shellfish for several days after heavy rains.
- Keep food refrigerated. The warmer it is, the less time it takes for food to reach temperatures that allow germs to grow and multiply.
- Keep rodents out of your home. Seal up any cracks and holes that would allow rodents to enter your home. Keep food in glass or hard plastic containers with tight-fitting lids. Keep kitchen and pet areas clean.

## Community Solutions

In addition to making changes in your personal life, you can work with your community to make these changes:

- Create habitat in your neighborhood that supports and nurtures native mosquito predators, such as dragonflies, toads and frogs, birds, and bats.
- Eliminate good egg-laying sites for Asian tiger mosquitoes. In urban areas, these mosquitoes breed wherever water collects, including bottles and cans on the ground, potted plant saucers, buckets, or old tires. Fish in ponds will eat the mosquito larvae. Use fine-mesh screens to cover openings to rain barrels. Bird baths can be treated with products containing *Bacillus thuringiensis israelensis* (Bt), a special bacteria that produces a toxin that kills only mosquito larvae and doesn't harm other insects or animals. Keep rain

gutters clean to eliminate standing water. Even a few drops of water can provide a good home for Asian tiger mosquitoes, which thrive in urban environments.

## Regional, National, and International Solutions

Some policies are more effective if they are made at the state, national, and international levels:

- Support policies to keep the public health system strong.
  - Maintain and enhance disease surveillance systems.
  - Develop early warning systems based on weather and climate data, which are thought to be useful in predicting outbreaks of cholera, malaria, meningitis, dengue fever, Japanese encephalitis, St. Louis encephalitis, and influenza.[33]
- Improve cooperation among governments to track and eradicate infectious diseases around the world.

# Chapter

## Food: Nature's Bounty Bashed

It's late Friday, the day before Max and his family are to arrive, and Maria is at the end of another long day spent dealing with her very sick, elderly patients at the hospital. Now she's at the grocery store to stock the pantry before her house fills with her latest round of guests, but she's facing an unexpected surprise. Many of the fruits, vegetables, and other foods she used to buy are in short supply or they are expensive, with a loaf of bread going for more than seven dollars, fresh tomatoes at 7 dollars a pound, and onions—a staple in her home—at 12 dollars for a three-pound bag. Meats are pricier than she's ever seen them too, and flour, margarine, snacks, and virtually everything else she puts in the cart are three to four times more expensive than they were what seemed like just months ago.

She opens her cell phone and calls Moravia at home to complain and to check on the kids.

"Mo, I'm here at the store, and the food prices are out of sight," she laments.

"I know," he says, "I know, since you've been making me do the shopping lately. I paid seven bucks just for a bag of potato chips last week. It's that amazing drought in California and the flooding in Florida that's doing it."

"Water problems, food problems," she says, shaking her head. She pulls a box of cereal out of the basket and double-checks the price. "The kids' favorite cereal, Crafty Capers, is selling for 11 dollars a box! That's criminal."

"Yeah, well, they love them so you've got to get them," Moravia says. "But with Max and Sula and their kids almost here, I'm not sure how we're going to manage all of the food and water and who knows what."

Maria is also wondering to herself: how are we going to manage? Then she sees a small sign near the front of the store that explains why food prices have crept ever higher in recent months. It mentions the drought and heat that are crippling large parts of the country, floods in other places, the high prices of fuel that are increasing food-shipping costs, and the damaging storms that have devastated crops around the world. There's some mention of government-subsidized flour prices and $CO_2$ as well, but Maria remembers Mo is on the line and stops reading.

"Sorry, Mo. Just reading something." Then she says in a tremulous voice, "Mo, how are Keisha and Zach today?" She doesn't hear the answer. She already knows. . . .

## PLANTS, CLIMATE CHANGE, AND OUR FOOD SUPPLY

Climate change and accompanying droughts, heat waves, and storms have already caused massive crop losses here in the United States. Increases in $CO_2$ will improve some crop yields, at least in the short term, but they will reduce many others. And climate variability will make it very difficult to predict just how much food will be available in the future.

Some examples to date: the upper Great Plains states of Nebraska, the Dakotas, Montana, and Wyoming reported temperatures of 118°F (48°C) in July and August of 2006. Moderate to severe droughts for several years before that left the soil parched, drained water reserves, and sealed the fate of many farmers and ranchers who had no harvest, sold their cattle at a loss, and got out of the business.

The record heat waves of 2006 also caused more than a billion dollars of damage to California's dairy industry. California experienced 20 straight days of temperatures higher than 100°F (38°C), including three days that topped 113°F (45°C). More than 25,000 cows dropped dead in the heat despite farmers' attempts to cool them with sprinklers and giant fans. The poultry industry was also hit hard, losing 700,000 birds to the heat, according to area newspapers.

Then, during the summer of 2007, while residents of the U.S. Southeast were hoping and praying for rain to ease the worst drought in their history, Texans and Oklahomans were being washed away by floods. The deluges claimed lives, destroyed homes, and caused more than half a billion dollars of crop damage.[1]

These are just a few local stories about food losses. The same story is playing out throughout the world. And it is all happening because global warming is changing our temperature and weather patterns. It turns out that it's not all bad, though. In 2006 and 2007, some places in the eastern portion of the U.S. great plains states were experiencing good growing seasons. These variable events are consistent with what scientists project for our future in a warmer world. More of the precipitation we receive will come in the form of heavy rains, leaving long stretches of dry days in between these rain events. Severe droughts will likely increase in frequency and intensity, temperatures will climb in some places and be lower in others, and in any one place there will be more climatic ups and downs that reduce the stability that crops and livestock need to thrive.

Although farmers and ranchers may be the first to suffer from rising temperatures, we all need to eat. And as very few of us actually grow our own food anymore, we will be at the mercy of global warming. As chaotic weather makes it more challenging to grow food, higher food prices are in store for everyone. This situation may be compounded by the fact that much of the food on our grocery store shelves comes from the San Joaquin valley in California. Dinner items for most Iowans, for instance, have traveled an average of 1,500 miles to reach their tables, and an average meal consists of ingredients from at least five different countries, according to a study from the Leopold Center for Sustainable Agriculture in Iowa.[2] We may feel the food-cost pinch even more if the places from which much of our food comes are slammed by climate chaos.

## HOW CROPS GROW

It's instructive to know how our food crops grow so we can understand what climate change will do to those patterns of growth—and to our diets. Plants turn sunlight into a form of energy that nourishes us. To do this, they absorb $CO_2$ from the air and use it in a complex process called photosynthesis that changes sunlight into chemical energy. Plants then use this energy to build their stems and leaves, and they release oxygen into the air as a by-product. This is a remarkably convenient system for us; without plants we simply could not live. Plants, in all their diversity, inhabit every continent, including Antarctica. They range from tiny beings that can only be seen with a microscope to trees that tower hundreds of feet into the air. And no matter where they live, some creature has adapted itself to eat them.

Because plants absorb $CO_2$ from the air to use in photosynthesis, some plants will actually do better with more $CO_2$ in the air—at least in the short term. In a matter of years, that advantage is expected to be overpowered by the detrimental effects on plants of global warming, such as higher temperatures, more droughts and floods, and greater problems with pests. Rice, soybeans, and wheat are among the plants expected to grow more quickly and vigorously in the short term with higher concentrations of $CO_2$ in the atmosphere. Interestingly, some plants, such as maize (corn) and sorghum, already absorb as much $CO_2$ from the atmosphere as they can use, so increasing the amount of $CO_2$ doesn't help them.[3]

## HEAT'S HARM TO CROPS

A hallmark of climate change is rising temperatures around the globe, and this heat will affect our crops. Each plant has a temperature range in which it can survive and flourish that is unique to its species. As temperatures increase, plants that are already growing at the upper end of this span will be the first to succumb. Initially they'll grow more slowly, be more vulnerable to disease, or perhaps produce fewer fruits or seeds. The small rise in the average global temperature that has already occurred between 1981 and 2002, about 0.75°F (0.4°C), has resulted in a global net loss of 40 million tons per year of wheat, corn, and barley. That's about $5 billion in crop losses.[4]

Warmer temperatures in the northeastern United States already have caused plants to behave differently, with apple trees and grapevines blooming about eight days earlier. Although this provides a longer growing period, there are risks. Some fruits, such as Concord grapes, cranberries, and some apples, require a minimum chilling period—of one to two months of temperatures consistently below 45°F (7.2°C)—to make fruit. With winter ending earlier, these fruits might not get that period.[5] Likewise, if plants flower before the bees and other insect pollinators are out and active, fruit crops will suffer. And farmers remind us that even though it may begin to warm up earlier in the spring, erratic weather means sudden cold spells are still likely. Late frosts can damage flowers and developing fruit.

But warmer temperatures won't be universal. Remember that global warming is causing climate chaos. Following California's episode of searing heat in the summer of 2006, the winter of 2006–2007 brought record-breaking low temperatures to southern California, endangering its $1 billion citrus industry.[6]

The U.S. Department of Agriculture created its most recent plant-hardiness zone map in 1990. Because global warming has already increased temperatures since then, and because a revised map is not forthcoming, the Arbor Day Foundation created a new map, using the most recent data available from 5,000 weather stations around the country. Many areas of the country jumped up a zone, meaning they are warmer than they used to be, and a few areas leaped two zones. A few areas actually dropped a zone, reinforcing the reason that scientists prefer to use the term *climate change* instead of *global warming*. You can see this new map on the Arbor Day Foundation's Web site at http://www.arborday.org.

## CLIMATE CHANGE AND PESTICIDE USE ON CROPS

In addition to the vagaries of temperature and rainfall, plants also will have to contend with changes in the insects and diseases that attack them. In general, insects develop more quickly in warmer temperatures. Longer growing seasons also mean that some insect pests have time to complete additional egg-laying cycles. Warmer winters may allow some pests, such as aphids, to survive the winter more successfully, getting a jump on the next growing season.[7] Moreover, insect pests are more likely to be mobile and can quickly expand their territory into areas where biological controls, such as predators or a plant's ability to secrete a chemical toxin to discourage consumption of its leaves, don't yet exist.[8]

Because climate change's influence on temperature and rainfall is expected to increase problems with crop pests, researchers have determined that pesticide use also will increase. As an example, one study of the effects of current rain and temperature variability showed that when rainfall increased by even 1 percent, pesticide use increased on all five crops studied, which are corn, cotton, potatoes, soybeans, and wheat. When temperature increased by 1 percent, pesticide use again rose on all the crops studied except wheat.[9]

Pesticides are products specially designed to kill insects, bacteria, and viruses that eat crops and reduce yields. Unfortunately, these chemicals are not only harmful for their targets, they're also toxic to humans, other animals, and beneficial insects that eat harmful insects or pollinate crops. Many pesticides are neurotoxins that damage the nervous systems of insects and other living organisms. Malathion, for example, sold in most garden and hardware stores and even some grocery stores, is moderately toxic to humans. Rotenone, extracted from certain plants and sometimes sold as a "natural" or "safe" pesticide, is extremely toxic to aquatic organisms and has been linked to Parkinson's disease in humans.[10] Still, if Rotenone can be kept out of waterways, it's preferable to malathion and the other petroleum-based pesticides because they can take a long time to break down in the environment.

We know that large doses of pesticides are extremely toxic to humans, and accidental poisoning can cause serious damage and death. There is substantial concern among physicians and researchers that children may be more vulnerable to the toxic effects of pesticides, and these substances might cause neurological damage in relatively low doses. Preliminary research done in California, for example, found that pregnant women living close to fields sprayed with certain pesticides had a slightly increased but measurable risk of producing children with autism.[11] We do know that children are more vulnerable to a variety of environmental toxins, and responses to these toxins can show up as developmental problems. Although we don't yet have good data to show direct cause-and-effect relationships, it still makes sense to limit children's exposure to pesticides.[12]

## SOIL, EROSION, AND CLIMATE CHANGE

Pesticides do more than just eliminate pests on crops (and increase our risk for harm). They get into the soil in which our crops grow and destroy its ability to nourish our crops. Soil contains a community of organisms that live there. These organisms perform the very necessary function of decomposing once-living material and releasing the nutrients into a form that plant roots can absorb and use to create our food. Most people are never aware of all this activity in the soil. An acre of good-quality topsoil contains on average a ton of earthworms and insects, more than a ton of fungi, and about a ton of bacteria, protozoa, and algae—more than three tons of living organisms that are working for all of us to provide food.[13] If you spray that soil with pesticides, much of the soil community is killed along with whatever insects above ground were being targeted.

To replace the pesticide-destroyed healthy soil, farmers have to add chemical fertilizers to feed the crops. Climate change will threaten the health of the soil even more by changing patterns of rainfall. There will be more droughts that dry out the soil and kill the living organisms in it. Then heavy rainfall events will wash away the soil—or erode it. The soil also will be baked by global warming's higher temperatures, which also kills the organisms that are so vital to food production.

Salt contamination of our soils is another climate-change risk. Like humans, most plants don't tolerate lots of salt in their diets. When sea levels rise, saltwater drowns land that was previously salt-free or had much lower salt concentrations. As sea levels rise, the salty water is also apt to swamp freshwater wells, which tend to be shallow in coastal areas. Once saltwater has contaminated well water, the water is of little use for drinking or irrigating crops. Salt contamination, though, can also result from less obvious sources. During storms, big waves will wash saltwater onto land that's a long way from the shore, and salt-laden winds will deposit salt on plants far inland. During Hurricane Katrina, waves of salt-water were pushed far into the coastal marshland, killing plants and contributing to the loss of more than 200 square miles of coastal wetlands. The chapter on ecosystems will go into more detail about how that happens and why we should care.

## PLANTS AND OZONE

Our crops will experience another insult from climate change. You may recall from the chapter on air quality that ozone is damaging to our lungs. It turns out that it's just as damaging to plants.[3] Ozone damages the cells inside a plant's leaves and reduces the photosynthesis that allows a plant to turn sunlight into energy. Moreover, when there is more ozone in the air, plants are less willing to open up the "breathing pores" on their leaves, reducing the amount of $CO_2$ they take in. Interestingly, the climate models have not accounted for these facts in their projections of how quickly $CO_2$ will accumulate in the atmosphere and how quickly temperatures will rise as a result.[14]

## AFTER PEAK OIL AND ITS EFFECT ON FOOD

With all this talk about the risks climate change will pose to our food supply, have you ever really thought about where some of the food in your kitchen actually comes from and how many steps it has been through to get to you? It's worth considering if we're going to eat well in our near future.

The current U.S. agricultural system needs huge amounts of fossil fuels. Fertilizers are made primarily from natural gas, the production of which has been declining here in the United States since 1970. Almost all pesticides are made from petroleum as a starting chemical. During the past 30 years, the number of large U.S. farms has increased. About two-thirds of all farms are now larger than 1,000 acres, and a quarter are larger than 10,000 acres.[15] Large farms require large pieces of farm equipment, generally diesel fueled, to accomplish what used to be done by smaller pieces of equipment, lots of people, and draft animals. Then the resulting produce is transported, primarily by truck, to a variety of processing plants where it is sorted and packaged for distribution all over the country. Produce that is destined to be processed into other products follows an even more circuitous route.

To get a handle on this, let's look at the example of tomato ketchup. The Swedish Institute for Food and Biotechnology did an in-depth analysis of this common foodstuff. It found that the tomatoes were grown in the Mediterranean region and shipped to Italy to be turned into tomato paste. The paste was then packed into large plastic bags that were produced in the Netherlands and shipped to Italy. The bags of paste were then placed into steel barrels and shipped to Sweden where they were unloaded at the ketchup factory. The paste was mixed with ingredients shipped to Sweden from an unknown number of other countries and packed into five-layer plastic bottles that had been produced in the United Kingdom or Sweden from materials manufactured in Japan, Italy, Belgium, the United States, and Denmark. For tomatoes to become bottled ketchup, more than 30 processing stages were required, and then there were at least 29 transportation stages, many from thousands of miles away.[16] Although our ketchup here in the United States doesn't come from Sweden, the process is probably quite similar. Many other products on our pantry shelves have comparable life stories.

Part of the problem with this scenario is that our Earth's crust contains a finite supply of petroleum. As discussed in chapter 2, the world's demand for oil has continued to rise every year, but the worldwide supply of petroleum has leveled off at about 84 million barrels per day since the middle of 2005, according to the U.S. Energy Information Administration. Despite efforts to locate new oil reserves, it's inevitable that the supply of oil will decline in the near future. With demand outstripping supply, oil prices will climb. Not only will it cost more to fill up your gas tank, the cost of the food we've become accustomed to also will climb. What about clementines from Spain in the fall, peppers from Peru in the winter, and grapes from Chile throughout the year? Americans have come to rely on having a ready supply of fresh fruits and vegetables available all year long—even when winter's cold prevents our local crop production. We've also come to expect to pay no more than 10 percent of our income for food, down from 20 percent in 1950.[17]

Our current food system has become so normal for us, it's hard to imagine how it could come to an end. Yet it's possible for our society to transition our food system into a more reasonable and sustainable system for the long term. And we might want to do so similarly to Cuba, which now may be a model for sustainable food production.[18] Cuba's move to sustainability, however, was abrupt. For the latter part of the last century, cheap oil from the Soviet Union fueled Cuba's agricultural system. When the Soviet Union collapsed in 1991, Cuba's supply of cheap oil abruptly came to an end. Without artificial fertilizers, pesticides, and diesel fuel to run farm machinery—all derived from fossil fuels—Cuba's food production experienced a sudden downturn.

The Cuban government realized it needed to take drastic action to save its population from starvation. It quickly broke up the large farms into small family and cooperative plots, relearned how to grow food organically, relocated many city dwellers (some voluntarily, others not) into the countryside to become farmers, encouraged citizens to plant gardens in every available backyard and rooftop in the cities, drastically cut meat consumption (again, not so voluntarily), and eventually transformed its food production system. During this forced transition time, Cubans suffered. The average Cuban adult lost 20 pounds. The result, however, is that now all Cubans have enough food, and very little fossil fuel is needed to produce it.[18]

Although it's unlikely our supply of fossil fuel will be cut off as abruptly as Cuba's was, prices will rise as demand outstrips supply. We've already seen evidence of this in 2007 and 2008. While the Cuban government is fundamentally different from the United States government, we can still learn from the Cuban experience. The first casualties of life in an oil-constrained world will be fresh fruits and vegetables flown in from faraway places. Eventually, most of our food will need to be produced far closer to where it is consumed. Moreover, food production will have to do without large quantities of fertilizers and pesticides derived from fossil fuels. This does not mean, however, that farming techniques must revert to the way things were done in 1900. In the past 100-plus years, we have learned a lot about the earth and life sciences. Improved knowledge of biology, hydrology, and botany, for example, will help to improve growing, watering, harvesting, and processing techniques. Nonetheless, the coming convergence of less fossil fuel and climate chaos will create enormous problems in providing the foods we eat.

## AQUATIC AND MARINE FOOD SUPPLY

Plants form the base of the food chain on land, but in the oceans phytoplankton occupy this special place. Phytoplankton are tiny organisms that perform much the same function as land plants: they turn the Sun's energy into chemical energy that they then use to sustain themselves and to reproduce. Their growth rate ultimately controls the number of living creatures that the oceans can support. Phytoplankton usually can't be seen without a microscope, but if enough are present a greenish tinge is visible in the water. They are eaten by slightly larger creatures, which are eaten by still larger creatures, and so forth up the food chain.

The basic materials that phytoplankton need are sunlight, water, and inorganic nutrients such as iron, nitrogen, phosphorus, and silicon.

Because they require sunlight, they can survive only in the very shallow layers of the oceans. In general, higher temperatures limit the growth of phytoplankton.[19,20] This doesn't bode well for a healthy marine food chain in a warmer world.

Unfortunately, that's not the only threat that climate change poses to the marine food supply. The oceans have absorbed about half of all the $CO_2$ that we've produced since the beginning of the industrial revolution. That's great for removing harmful $CO_2$ from the atmosphere, but when $CO_2$ dissolves in water, carbonic acid is formed. As a result, the oceans are becoming more acidic. As you might guess, ocean creatures can survive in a very narrow range of acidity. Creatures that rely on shells to protect them from predators also will find themselves without a safe home because the calcium carbonate that forms their shells breaks down in more acidic water, softening the shell and making the creature inside vulnerable to being eaten.[21]

These small creatures tend to occupy relatively low positions in the marine food chain, meaning that anything that affects *their* well-being will also affect the well-being of everything above them. Although the marine animals that rely on a diet of shellfish might initially be well fed because their chosen prey will have no defense, the shellfish will quickly be wiped out and then their predators will be in a pickle. Shellfish predators, such as the octopus, the starfish, and some crabs and fish, will have difficulty surviving without the shellfish. Other fish, eels, and dolphins that normally dine on octopus, for example, will then find themselves without their usual food supply. This devastating process works its way up the food chain.

Add to this feature of climate change the serious mismanagement of ocean fisheries and the marine ecosystem, and you might realize its effects on us. And although farmed fish may seem like a reasonable alternative to wild caught fish, most fish farms do more damage to wild fish populations than you might think. Because most fish are carnivorous, farmed fish must be fed up to four pounds of wild-caught fish for every pound of farmed fish harvested. Moreover, fish farms have devastated wild fish habitat in some areas.[22]

## CLIMATE CHANGE AND FOOD TOXINS

The consequences of a changing climate hold many other surprises in store for us. One of those surprises recently came to light when researchers discovered that certain toxins, such as mercury, could increase in our food supply as a result of global warming.

Most of the mercury currently in our diets comes from the burning of coal for electric power. This process begins when small amounts of mercury, found naturally in coal, are released into the atmosphere as the coal is burned. The mercury then settles into the soil, washes into our waterways when it rains, and is turned into a more lethal form by bacteria before fish take it up. We eat those fish and ingest the mercury. This process is enhanced as the water becomes more acidic, often from power plants' sulfur emissions that cause "acid rain," and now also as the oceans become more acidic from absorbing $CO_2$. In addition, as water is diverted from streams and lakes for large hydroelectric projects, more mercury is concentrated in the remaining water and in the fish.[23] Peat bogs also contain high concentrations of mercury, which isn't much of a problem as long as the mercury stays in the bogs. Unfortunately, the warming world is causing peat bogs to burn more frequently, and their mercury is also released into the air, following the same path into our fish.[24]

Mercury, like all heavy metals, is not broken down in the body. Instead, it *bioaccumulates*. As small fish, with small amounts of mercury in their bodies, are eaten by larger fish, the mercury accumulates in the larger fish. The larger fish get eaten by still larger fish, and the mercury concentration just keeps increasing. Eventually, humans consume the big fish and unwittingly get all the mercury that had accumulated in the fish.

Mercury worsens the harm climate change causes because it is a dangerous toxin that injures human brains and nervous systems, especially in developing fetuses, babies, and young children but also in adults. It results in lowered intellect and behavior changes in children. In adults, it can lead to heart disease and an increased risk of heart attack at fairly low doses. A study of Wisconsin men and women found that men had higher mercury levels than women who consumed the same amount of fish, so men may be at higher risk of heart attack from mercury consumption.[25] Although mercury is extremely toxic, perhaps the greatest concern is the other nasty surprises that likely are in store for us if we don't get our climate stabilized. The story of mercury and its travels also illustrates that solutions to reducing greenhouse gases—by reducing the amount of coal used to produce electricity—have many other benefits to our health by reducing air pollution and minimizing mercury in the environment and in our diets.

## HOW MUCH OF AN EFFECT?

Given all of the repercussions climate change will have on our food production, current predictions estimate that overall global food production will only suffer about 15 percent, although this does not account for the local and regional variation in food production.[26] Farmers in the

United States, for example, may not be able to continue growing the same crops, potentially leading to their financial ruin before they receive the help they need to learn new techniques. They may have to learn how to grow different crops and acquire new equipment, such as drip irrigation systems, to produce crops with much less water. Although making these changes will be painful for those involved, these changes could be disastrous in other parts of the world.

Bangladesh, for example, is a crowded country in which climate change will severely compromise the country's ability to produce food. India, with about a sixth of the world's population, could experience as much as a 40 percent reduction in food production, primarily from changes in temperature and rainfall. On the other hand, Russia is looking forward to increased grain production as some of its frozen land thaws out.[26] In general, countries in the northern latitudes may see increased crop production, although farmers likely will need to adapt to new crops and growing techniques. Whether it will be enough to make up for the losses farther south, and whether affordable means of transporting crops can be found in an age of shrinking oil supplies, remains to be seen. Growing inequities between the rich and the poor are a likely result.

## MEAT: WHAT WE EAT DRIVES CLIMATE CHANGE

Now that we've reviewed how climate change will affect our food supply, let's turn the tables and look at how what we eat contributes to climate change. Livestock contribute about one-fifth of all greenhouse emissions globally. That's as much as the transportation sector! In addition, livestock use about a fourth of our available supplies of fresh water. In 2006, the United Nations Food and Agriculture Organization (FAO) produced a 400-page report documenting all the ways that raising livestock leads to climate change. Globally, meat, dairy, and eggs provide about one-third of all dietary protein, and the global production of meat is expected to double by 2050. This figure, however, belies the harsh differences in meat consumption between countries. For example, one Indian eats an annual average of 11 pounds (5 kg) of meat compared to the average American who consumes 270 pounds (123 kg) a year.[27] Livestock must be fed, requiring much land for grazing and to grow crops for animal feed. In fact, the FAO reports that the land used to raise livestock is the largest of all human land uses, requiring forests to be constantly cleared for pastureland use in some regions. Cattle ranching is now the main reason for deforestation in the

Amazon. In other regions, overgrazing or grazing on marginal lands has caused deserts to grow and spread, swallowing entire towns and further compromising the ability of people to grow food. By 2050, global population is expected to increase by about 40 percent and global meat consumption is expected to double, primarily in low- and middle-income countries, producing a disastrous further increase in greenhouse gas emissions.

Dr. Anthony McMichael, one of the world's foremost authorities on the health effects of climate change, has worked with his colleagues to calculate how much global meat production should be reduced to prevent increased greenhouse gas emissions. They acknowledge that some societies consume more meat than is healthy, contributing to obesity and a variety of chronic diseases, whereas other societies could benefit nutritionally from more meat and animal protein in their diets. They recommend that the average daily consumption of meat be reduced slightly from the current amount of 3.5 ounces (100 g) to 3.1 ounces (90 g) and that less than half of that amount should come from red meat. (Cattle, sheep, and goats, common "red-meat" animals, have multiple stomachs and produce a lot more methane, which contributes to global warming, as part of their normal digestive process.) Meeting these recommendations would require, however, a significant redistribution in who eats meat and how much of it they eat. The average American would need to reduce meat consumption by about 75 percent from a daily average of 12 ounces to 3.1 ounces, while the average Indian would need to increase consumption of daily meat by almost six times to reach the 3.1-ounce target.[28]

## OTHER CONTRIBUTORS TO CLIMATE CHANGE

Other food-related activities that contribute to climate change include applying too much nitrogen fertilizer to the soil, which allows some of it to aerosolize and become a greenhouse gas about 300 times more potent than $CO_2$ for warming the Earth. Digging or tilling the soil also allows the carbon that has been stored there to be released into the atmosphere. Perhaps the most damaging practice is our collective lust for cheap ingredients grown in the tropics. The low price of palm oil has made it a ubiquitous component of practically every kind of packaged food as well as many personal-care and cleaning products. Increasing demand has led to tropical forests being cleared and peat bogs being drained to plant more palm oil trees, releasing a lot of carbon into the atmosphere. Because palm oil is also in demand as a starting ingredient for biodiesel, we will discuss this in the following section.

## BIOFUELS

*Biofuel*, a term used to describe any biological matter that is used for fuel, was the only source of fuel until humans figured out how to extract and use fossil fuels. In addition to burning wood, crop residues, or even cow dung for fuel, biofuel also now refers to converting plant matter into liquid fuels such as ethanol and biodiesel. Theoretically, using biofuels to replace gasoline or diesel made from fossil fuels could significantly reduce greenhouse gas emissions. The $CO_2$ released from the burning of raw biofuels equals the carbon the plant matter absorbed from the atmosphere during its lifetime, so there would theoretically be a climate-change "wash." Stuffing a few branches into your gas tank and lighting them on fire, however, is unlikely to help you get to work. To convert plant matter to ethanol requires the addition of energy, which is currently supplied by fossil fuels. Not all plant matter is created equal in terms of its ethanol potential. The primary source of ethanol currently used in the United States is corn. Corn, it turns out, is one of the least efficient starters for ethanol.

Proponents of corn-based ethanol claim that about 30 percent more energy is released when corn ethanol is burned than the amount of energy that went into creating the ethanol, and greenhouse gas emissions are about 18 percent less than conventional gasoline.[29,30] Although that sounds like an improvement, other researchers claim that it doesn't tell the whole story.

As we saw during 2007, corn prices hit record highs as a result of increased demand from the ethanol refineries. The high price of corn, in turn, drove up prices of meat and milk because corn is a major component in animal feed. As farmers were able to make more money growing corn for ethanol, farmland that had previously been planted in other crops was planted in corn instead, causing relative shortages of other cereal crops and driving up their prices, too. A growing number of researchers say, however, that even this expanded view of the effects of turning corn into liquid fuel doesn't tell the whole story.

Recent studies indicate that how we use a piece of land—whether it's to grow a fuel crop such as corn to reduce the amount of fossil fuels used or to grow trees to absorb carbon—makes a huge difference in the carbon balance of the Earth. Forestation of the land would absorb and store up to nine times more carbon over a 30-year period than the carbon reduction benefits achieved by burning the gasoline-replacing ethanol made from that land! The same researchers also calculated that to substitute just 10 percent of our present gasoline and diesel use with biofuels would require 43 percent—almost half—of all current cropland in the United States. If we intend to continue to feed our population, we would need to clear a lot more land to grow the fuel crops, and clearing the land of its prairie or forest would result in that much more carbon released to the atmosphere. These researchers conclude that it would make more sense to focus on improving the efficiency of fossil fuel use while conserving existing forests and prairies and converting any cropland that's not needed for food to forest or prairie to absorb additional $CO_2$.[31]

Other researchers compared a variety of biofuels and concluded that only those produced from waste products, such as used cooking oil, methane from manure, or ethanol from grass or wood, were better for overall climate stabilization than gasoline. The absolute worst biofuels for the climate are U.S.-produced corn ethanol, Brazil-produced ethanol made from sugarcane, biodiesel made from soy, and Malaysian biodiesel made from palm oil.[32]

Already 1 billion people, or about one-sixth of the world's population, go hungry, and 5 million children starve to death every year. It becomes morally difficult to justify using food crops to fill gasoline tanks instead of stomachs. *Cellulosic ethanol*, however, is a new technology that creates ethanol from woody material instead of a food crop through a chemical process using an acid. Switchgrass, a tall prairie grass, or perhaps trees grown on marginal land that can't be used for farming, are potential starters for cellulosic ethanol production. The technology to produce cellulosic ethanol is not yet commercially viable, but it could be in the near future.

## CLIMATE, FOOD, AND MENTAL HEALTH

Given all the concerns about the relationship between climate change and our food supply, it's essential to note that it is not only our health that could be harmed. Inadequate nutrition also is associated with many developmental and behavioral problems in children, including lower IQs.[33,34] Inadequate access to food resources also increases the risk for serious mental health and coping problems.[35,36] Importantly, socioeconomic disadvantage already is one of the primary reasons for malnutrition, and climate change would exacerbate this problem for the world's poor people.[37]

There is an additional concern about food resources. The very lack of sufficient food for good health and mental functioning creates what is called food insecurity. Although little research into food insecurity and mental health has been done, it appears that people exposed to food and water shortages may be more traumatized as a result.[35] Food insecurity may increase the risk of depression and anxiety, including post-traumatic stress disorder, as was described in several other chapters. Moreover, food insecurity also appears to be associated with women experiencing higher risks of violence and mental suffering.[38] Food shortages plainly may contribute to more interpersonal conflict.

Pesticides have their own possible harmful effects on child development and our mental functioning. Although the research remains limited, scientists caution that developmental disabilities, neurological problems, depression, anxiety, and other psychological and behavioral conditions may result from pesticide exposure.[39–41] So the potential for climate change to create more nutritional deprivation, food insecurity, and pesticide exposure, especially among children and other vulnerable people, may alone create enormous mental health crises around the world.

## SOLUTIONS

### Individual Solutions

You can reduce the risks that global warming poses to your diet and prevent food-related climate change by taking some basic steps:

- Buy locally produced organic food when possible.
- Get to know the producers of your food by buying from a farmer's market or community-supported agriculture. Seek producers who control pests without pesticides and use organic methods to fertilize rather than petroleum-based fertilizers.
- Wash your fruits and vegetables well.
- Try growing some of your own food. That way you'll know exactly what went into the soil and what pesticides or fertilizers were used, if any. This may also help to shield your family from rising fuel costs and provide a stronger connection to your environment. A multitude of resources, both online and from the library or bookstore, are available to help you be a successful organic gardener. *Organic Gardening* is a how-to magazine filled with lots of practical tips.
- Eat less meat—and a lot less red meat. Meat production requires more resources than the same amount of calories from plant sources. Meatless Monday is a national campaign to help people reduce their meat

consumption starting with just one day a week. Many larger businesses and schools have signed on to provide a meat-free lunch option on Mondays. The three-ounce daily portion recommended earlier in the chapter is about the size of an average hamburger patty. There are health and environmental benefits to eating even less meat—or no meat at all. When you do eat meat, try to purchase locally produced meat from pasture-fed animals that were raised without antibiotics in their feed.

- If you eat fish, choose varieties that are sustainably fished. Several organizations offer lists of fish to avoid due to high mercury contamination or unsustainable fishing practices.
- Compost your food waste to reduce methane emissions and filling up landfills. The compost adds valuable organic matter to soil in gardens and landscaping. Information about how to compost can be found on *Organic Gardening* magazine's Web site as well as on many others.

## Community Solutions

At the community level:

- Encourage more farmer's markets in your community.
- Encourage local restaurants and grocery stores to buy more organic and locally grown produce.
- Get involved with land-use planning:
  - Reduce the numbers of fast-food chains. They serve mostly meat, and the food typically comes from central processing plants, hindering local procurement and requiring the food to travel long distances.
  - Make sure all neighborhoods in your city have access to a grocery store with good-quality fresh produce.
- Get involved with local schools and school boards to encourage the use of more locally grown, organic, fresh produce in school lunches.

## Regional, National, and International Solutions

- Let your policy makers know that you support the Treaty of the Seas to limit catches in international waters. This treaty would allow fish populations that have been overfished to recuperate.
- Support cap-and-trade systems for nutrients. These systems limit the amounts of fertilizers, especially nitrogen, that can be used, keeping excess nitrogen out of waterways and the atmosphere. Nitrogen adds to the dead zones in coastal waters. More about that in the chapter on ecosystems.

- Encourage your policy makers to offer incentives for local organic-food production wherever possible and punishments to discourage bad practices
  that add to global warming or are unsustainable.
- Discourage the use of corn-based ethanol as an alternative to fossil fuels.
  Instead, encourage improved efficiency to reduce the amount of fossil fuels
  used and to switch to clean, renewable energy sources.

# Chapter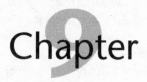

## Ecosystem Health:
## Cycles of Life . . . Or Death

The clock chimes 11 times the night before Max and his family are to arrive. The house is quiet, but then Zach's coughing spell disrupts the silence. Maria catches her breath, waiting apprehensively for the coughing to stop. It does, and she relaxes and looks down again at the book she's been paging through.

It's one of those old coffee-table books from her childhood filled with gorgeous photographs of the natural world. She's overcome by sadness that her children will never see many of these remarkable sights. She tries to understand—she needs to understand—how it all fits together.

The Earth has been warming for years. She knows this. Global warming is a household term now. Everything is blamed on global warming these days. Yet how could only a few degrees of warming cause so much harm?

She lingers over a photo of the rolling prairies not far from her home. Once wheat, rye, and barley grew easily there. She remembers seeing hundreds of ducks on the prairie wetlands, too. But water has become scarce as the storms and rain have become more variable. Yes, sometimes there are strange spates of brutal storms now—just a week ago six tornadoes and massive downpours destroyed two small towns 60 miles away—only to have extended droughts descend. With the ancient underground water supply almost gone, many of the fields stand parched and empty. Feed for livestock is tremendously expensive, making meat extremely overpriced. And water restrictions are the norm.

Maria flips the page and sees a photo of a vast river—gently serpentine, brimming with water, the nation's waterway. Except she drives over it every day going to and from work at the hospital, and now it's rarely larger than a stream. Not enough water for our crops to drink either, Maria thinks. We're importing more food from elsewhere to compensate. No wonder food is so expensive.

A few photos later show vast forests along the flanks of snow-capped mountains where her sister Magda once lived. The caption says "Rocky Mountain National Park." She remembers visiting that park as a child on a family vacation. Even then many of the trees were dead because they had been weakened from declining snow and rainfall, the very moisture that once filled our rivers and streams. In their weakened state, the trees ultimately fell prey to a tree-eating bug that climate change allowed to climb higher as the warming temperatures expanded the insect's range.

Maria thinks, with the dead prairies and the dead trees from bugs and not enough consistent moisture—and all of the rain forests almost gone around the world, too—we just don't have the plants anymore to deal with the $CO_2$ we keep putting into the atmosphere. We're getting warmer by the day.

She is beginning to see the natural interconnections in the world around her, but the beautiful photos call her back. She flips to a broad aerial photo of a coastal wetland where her once-great river spills into the Gulf of Mexico. In the picture, the city of New Orleans is evident to one side. Maria knows it's mostly an abandoned town now, what with the rising sea levels from the melting ice caps and the series of hurricanes swamping it one too many times. A smaller inset photo shows an oil rig out in the gulf, and Maria laughs to think how gasoline is so expensive now and mostly used by pharmaceutical companies to make medicines. Synthetic fuels made from coal and plants—ridiculously expensive now, too—power cars these days. Yet she knows that these fuels continue to push more and more $CO_2$ into the atmosphere.

The next few photos show an undersea life in the gulf and the oceans that simply doesn't exist anymore. She sees schools of brightly colored fish swimming through purple and green sea fans, orange sponges, and slender branches of red coral. The warming temperatures have killed much of the coral, which once sheltered many types of juvenile fish. And the seas have become too acidic, killing off even more underwater life, because they have been absorbing a lot of the $CO_2$ that humans keep churning out.

Maria winces at one of the next photos, another small inset. It shows a fishing trawler in the gulf that had just brought up a huge amount of fish and other sea creatures using an enormous net. She hadn't really thought about why there are rarely fish available in the grocery store any more.

And she says to herself, hanging her head in weariness, "I've never really thought about where everything comes from and how everything on Earth is interconnected. We've been destroying all of the pieces, the web of life, bit by bit."

She flips randomly through the old photos now, and she can see how climate change has amplified other destructive human actions. What remains of the forests is dying. The plains are parched. Water and food supplies are stretched thin, and they are ever more expensive. The air is bad. Storms come in waves and do great harm, but they don't replenish the water. The seas are practically empty. People are sicker and more stressed than ever before. It's all connected. But where do we start to get things back to the way they were? The clock begins to chime again, and Maria is startled out of her thoughts. Max and his family will be here tomorrow—today. "We'll manage," she thinks. "We'll have to."

## ECOSYSTEMS AND OUR HEALTH

Maria's dawning realization that climate change harms all of life is the grist for this chapter. When our ecosystems are compromised, they are no longer able to offer us the "services"—clean air, plentiful water, decent food, and more—that we rely on for our health and well-being. And we have yet to find technological substitutes for these necessities.

Our activities already have deeply stressed many of Earth's ecosystems. We've polluted our water, soil, and air. We've logged and extracted other resources, harming the land. We've fragmented habitats through our suburban development and growth. We've diverted, dammed, and drained our waterways to drink, water our lawns, and irrigate our crops. We've exterminated many animal and plant species, destroying biodiversity. Climate change is turning out to be a colossal stress with the potential to push some of our ecosystems beyond hope of adaptation and into actual collapse.

We've already talked about some of the basic ecosystem services. Other healthy ecosystem services include adequate soil fertility; raw materials for constructing shelter, clothing, or medicines; natural pest control; buffering from storms; and the provision of a stable climate.

### Farms and Prairies

Maria first notes what hits closest to home for her. Fertile prairies and farms could transform into drier scrub-type vegetation if we continue to pump $CO_2$ into the atmosphere and temperatures climb. Higher concentrations of $CO_2$ over the prairies cause a 20-fold increase in the growth of woody shrubs, which crowd out prairie grasses and provide less suitable habitat for livestock.[1] In Chapter 5, we mentioned the ancient waters of the Ogallala aquifer, which currently provide much of the irrigation water for the western region of the U.S. Midwest, and learned that the aquifer will not be able to provide current levels of water for much longer. It's simply not getting recharged, and climate change will deepen that reality with more droughts and water shortages.

In the central region of North America, lying across the U.S.–Canada border, a prairie wetland provides such critical ecosystem services as groundwater recharge, water for agriculture, and water purification. Called the Prairie Pothole Region, this area is famous as "the duck factory of North America," producing more than half of North America's ducks by some estimates. Long-term monitoring of the Prairie Pothole Region's climate shows that noticeable changes are already occurring: The western part of the region is getting drier, and the eastern part is getting wetter. Future climate projections for this area indicate milder winters as well as warmer, longer, and drier summers. Although the eastern portion may get more moisture, warmer temperatures and higher evaporation rates may counteract the greater amounts of moisture. Moreover, more than 95 percent of the eastern wetlands have been drained for agriculture. Only restoration of wetlands and nesting habitat in the eastern part could help to offset some of the drying in the west so that the Prairie Pothole Region could continue to produce waterfowl in wetter years.[2]

## Mountains

Water for the prairie heartland comes from a number of sources, including the wetlands and the Ogallala aquifer. It also comes from the Rocky Mountains. The snowpack there melts slowly through the summer and, when it is plentiful, it provides steady water supplies to many rivers and streams in North America. With the warmer temperatures that accompany climate change, more of the mountain precipitation is projected to come as rainfall instead of snow, depriving waterways of water throughout the summer when the water is most needed. Maria sees this in the shrinking rivers near her home. It's little consolation that the loss of forest and plant cover in the mountains will lead to more water runoff after the heavier storms that are expected. Rivers may then briefly flood, but with less water soaking into the ground to be naturally purified and to recharge underground water sources, more of the water that does end up downstream is apt to be polluted.

## Forests and Biodiversity

Maria recalls the bug- and drought-induced devastation to the mountain forests. Climate change's damage to our forests in the mountains and across the planet will cause more than just the loss of clean water. A healthy forest ecosystem requires *biodiversity*, or a variety of different life forms, to function. Loss of biodiversity is affecting practically all of Earth's ecosystems, but some more than others.

It may not be obvious, for example, why we should care about mosquitoes in the jungle far away from us. If we didn't know their function there before, why should we care if they're eradicated? You also may not be aware of a small collection of cells located in your pancreas called the Islets of Langerhans, but without them you would develop diabetes. In the same way, we often don't know the vital role a species may play in the overall functioning of an ecosystem until it's gone. Only then do we see the harm that results.

So let's tell the tale of these mosquitoes. In the 1950s, health officials in the tropical forests of Borneo tried to reduce malaria rates by spraying an insecticide to kill the mosquitoes. Many of them died, and malaria rates decreased—but then something curious happened. The geckos and lizards that ate the mosquitoes began dying, partly because they didn't have enough of their favored mosquitoes to eat and possibly because they ingested some poison when they did eat a few. Then the wildcats that ate the geckos and lizards died. Without the cats, there was an explosion of rats in the village. Rats carry fleas, which carry the disease typhus. Spraying the insecticide to kill the mosquitoes ended up decreasing malaria rates for a while, but it resulted in a typhus epidemic among the people.

Picture that mosquito ecosystem as a spider's web with each node of the web representing the various interconnected species. The service the web provides for the spider is to catch food. If we remove just one of the nodes—take the mosquitoes out of our ecosystem—there's a good chance the web will continue to function fairly well to catch other insects for the spider to eat. But if removing the mosquitoes results in many holes in the web—because of the interdependencies of insects in combination with such ecosystem assaults as pollution, loss of habitat, or global warming—eventually the web will become so full of holes that it can no longer provide the service of catching food for the spider.

In general, we don't know much yet about the intricacies of many ecosystems and their biodiversity. We tend to learn about how important a particular species was to the functioning of the ecosystem when it becomes rare or extinct and we see the consequences. We have learned, however, that in many ecosystems there are certain key species that are critical to the ecosystems' continued functioning. In our spider web analogy, these key species would be represented by structurally important nodes of the web—maybe those that hold the web in place. If these species become rare or extinct, the web could collapse, even if most of the other species are still present.

We've already mentioned an example of this in the higher altitudes of the Rocky Mountains. Since the 1970s, the Rocky Mountains have warmed 2°F (1.1°C). That's apparently enough for the pine beetle to extend its range into the higher elevations where whitebark pines are the dominant tree species. Although these trees have no commercial value, their seeds feed squirrels, many kinds of birds, and grizzly bears in the fall, allowing the necessary fat accumulation that will get the bears through the winter. As the whitebark pines are weakened by drought and warmer temperatures and succumb to the beetles, the fate of the birds and animals that rely on the pine seeds—especially the grizzlies—is unknown. [3]

## COASTAL WETLAND ECOSYSTEMS AND STORM BUFFERS

Our coastal ecosystems also provide vital ecosystem services to us, as Maria saw in the photos. Most important, they buffer the land from storms and give us vital food resources. Sadly, along the coast of the Gulf of Mexico the integrity of the coastal ecosystem has been severely compromised by loss of land, an invasive species consuming wetland plants, and accelerated erosion from the oil and gas industry. Climate change is adding to these destructive factors there and elsewhere around the world.

In 1940, the U.S. Corps of Army Engineers began a massive project to contain the powerful waters of the Mississippi River and prevent the periodic flooding that damaged towns and farmlands. Through a series of dams and levees, the Corps eventually tamed the Mighty Mississippi, but not without consequences for the coastal ecosystem. Without the silt that was carried down from northern lands and deposited at the mouth of the river to build up new coastal land to replace what was naturally worn away by erosion, the coast began losing land mass. This process was enhanced by thousands of miles of canals that were dug to facilitate the extraction of oil and natural gas from the Gulf of Mexico. The canals provide the basis for enhanced erosion, resulting in additional land loss—nearly 1,500 square miles (4,000 km$^2$) of Louisiana coastal wetlands have been lost since 1940.

Another major blow to the coastal ecosystem came from a small, furry creature called a nutria. This creature was introduced from South

America in the 1930s to stimulate fur trade in the area. Apparently, Americans didn't find the prospect of nutria fur coats as appealing as the nutria found the tasty marsh plants of their new home. With very few natural enemies, these creatures munched their way through acres of land-holding marsh plants, adding to the erosion problem.

As the buffering of the coastal wetlands gradually has been lost, storms have done even more damage and eroded the coastline far more quickly than before. Usually, between 25 and 50 square miles are lost every year. Hurricane Katrina, however, caused the direct loss of more than 200 square miles of coastal land and was indirectly responsible for even more lost acreage as the storm surge pushed salt water far into the marsh. The salt contaminated the soil, causing the slow poisoning of more coastal habitat.

That surge, moreover, helped to turn large swathes of living trees that had been absorbing and storing carbon before the storm into dead and rotting trees that then released their stored carbon back into the atmosphere. As we discussed in Chapter 2, living trees and plants are excellent "carbon sinks" that the storms associated with climate change will increasingly destroy, demonstrating another one of those positive feedback loops that aren't too positive for our health and well-being.[4]

Finally, our coastal ecosystems do more than provide us with important food. The marshy Gulf Coast, for example, produces about one-third of the nation's seafood, worth $3 billion per year. This habitat also provides another important ecosystem service as the winter feeding grounds for most of the migratory waterfowl in North America, and it's the first place many of these birds can rest and eat after flying 500 miles nonstop across the Gulf of Mexico. Without this habitat, we might lose even more of our vital ecosystem biodiversity.

## Marine Ecosystems

Just off our coasts, warmer temperatures also are occurring in the sea, and coral reefs are especially sensitive. Most coral reefs currently exist at the upper end of their acceptable temperature range, so it won't take much additional warming to push them over the edge into a range they can no longer tolerate. Coral reefs are underwater gardens of a vast array of species that can't live anywhere else. In fact, many coral reefs are home to some of the greatest biodiversity on Earth. In addition to their permanent residents, coral reefs offer nursery habitat for many fishes and other sea creatures that will live most of their lives in open water when they get big enough to survive on their own. In this way, the loss of coral reefs from rising temperatures also will have a tremendous impact on open-water species. Global warming, however, is not the only factor threatening the survival of many fish species.

The oceans are so vast and foreign to many, it may seem like there's no end to the fish and sea creatures that live beneath the surface. But as Maria saw in the fishing trawler net, overfishing has taken a greater toll on the health of marine ecosystems than many people realize. As of 2003, almost 30 percent of all fisheries had collapsed (meaning that the recorded catches of those fish species are less than 10 percent of the recorded maximums). There simply aren't enough of those fish species left to continue fishing them, according to a team of 14 scientists from five countries that looked at overfishing and biodiversity loss. In fact, despite more fishing boats, more fishermen, and better fishing technology globally, total catches of all commercial fish species have decreased by 13 percent from the maximum catches that occurred in 1994. If current overfishing pressures continue, scientists estimate that all the marine life that humans harvest will be gone by 2048, leaving hundreds of millions of people without their main protein source.[5]

## Marine Dead Zones

Still another threat to marine ecosystems comes from a seemingly paradoxical circumstance. In the Gulf of Mexico along the Louisiana and Mississippi coast, there is a vast area that doesn't support life. The reason for this "dead zone" and others around the world is an overabundance of nutrients, which sounds like it ought to be a good thing. It isn't. These nutrients, mostly fertilizers from farm runoff, such as nitrogen, phosphorus, and potassium, have tripled in volume since about 1960. The nutrients stimulate the growth of algae, which then use up all the oxygen in the water, leaving the rest of the ocean in that area without enough oxygen to support life. The size of the dead zone varies each summer, depending mainly on how much flooding occurred in the Midwest (flooding washes more nutrients into the Gulf), how much of these nutrients were applied to farms in the Midwest, and the presence of stormy conditions in the Gulf of Mexico that stir up the water and improve the oxygen content. So far, the largest dead zones were seen in 2001, 2002, and 2007; in these years, the dead zone was about as large as the state of New Jersey.[6] Another dead zone recently turned up in the Pacific Ocean off the coast of Oregon, and dead zones also typically occur in the Chesapeake Bay, Lake Erie, and in more than 140 other waters worldwide. There is concern now that climate change, through changing wind and ocean currents, could result in more of these dead zones—separate from those caused by farm nutrient runoff.[7]

In the chapter on food, we already discussed how warmer temperatures are harming the phytoplankton, the "plants of the sea," and how $CO_2$ absorption is leading to the seawater becoming more acidic and preventing the shell formation of sea creatures. When those food chain pressures on marine life survival are combined with critical overfishing, warmer temperatures that kill off coral reefs, and expanding dead zones, the result is a marine ecosystem in serious trouble. Restoring the health of the marine ecosystem is absolutely critical to maintaining the health of human populations.

## BIODIVERSITY LOSS AND INFECTIOUS DISEASE

The climate-fueled loss of our marine ecosystems and the nourishment they provide to us; the loss of our coastal protections; and the losses to our forests, farms, water resources, and air quality all will have an impact on our health and well-being. We haven't the space to describe the myriad interconnections in this weakening biodiversity web, but let's circle back to Lyme disease as one example.

Lyme disease, mentioned briefly in the chapter on infectious diseases, is caused by bacteria that are transmitted by the deer tick (*Ixodes scapularis*). Deer tick larvae (tick babies) require a blood meal before becoming nymphs (tick adolescents), which then require another blood meal before maturing into adults and reproducing. Despite their name, deer ticks are willing to take their blood meal from any creature that has blood—reptiles, amphibians, birds, or mammals.

If the Lyme disease bacteria are present in the area and there is a good biodiversity of animals in the tick's habitat, the tick can get its blood meal from all manner of creatures. This means it has only a 30 percent chance of biting an animal that is infected with Lyme disease and ingesting the bacteria into its own little body. If, however, there has been loss of biodiversity from suburban sprawl or the habitat fragmentation that has driven out many of our larger mammals, the tick has a greater chance of getting its blood meal from the ubiquitous white-footed mouse, which only requires small parcels of habitat for survival. The white-footed mouse is especially good at carrying Lyme disease.

Research shows that as wooded habitat shrinks, there is less biodiversity but a greater density of white-footed mice. If a tick bites a white-footed mouse in the U.S. Northeast and Mid-Atlantic states where Lyme disease bacteria are common, it has an 80 percent chance of getting infected with Lyme disease. In areas that have more intact woodland with good biodiversity, the effect is "diluted" because there are so many more options for the tick to get its blood meal. So loss of biodiversity leads to an increased risk of Lyme disease for us. Conversely, maintaining good animal and forest biodiversity can reduce the risk of humans contracting Lyme disease.[8] This situation is but one example of how biodiversity loss can increase our risk for infectious disease.

## BIODIVERSITY LOSS = EXTINCTION

Human activities already have caused the extinction of between 5 and 20 percent of species on Earth; and as many as 50 percent of currently living species may be extinct by 2050 if we continue to destroy critical habitat and allow global warming to continue unabated.[9] The loss of so many species—current rates of extinction are estimated to be up to 1,000 times greater than before humans walked the Earth—will have grave consequences for our ecosystems as well as for human society. The loss of biodiversity, including creatures and plants we don't even know about, will undoubtedly result in both economic and health risks.

As our ecosystems become degraded and some plants become extinct from the effects of climate change and human activity, the ability of those ecosystems to serve as $CO_2$ sinks is also degraded. When they can no longer continue to absorb 50 percent of all $CO_2$ emissions as they do now, more of our emissions will go into the atmosphere, making the potential for abrupt and potentially catastrophic climate change more likely. If we continue on our present path, estimates indicate that by the end of the century the sinks will be so degraded that they will hardly be able to absorb any additional $CO_2$ at all.[10] Researchers from Europe have found evidence that degradation of the land sink has likely already begun. They say that sharp increases in atmospheric $CO_2$ since 2000 are consistent with less $CO_2$ uptake by plants, primarily due to widespread drought. This could mean that we are rapidly approaching or have passed a key tipping point in the climate system.[11] Thus, healthy ecosystems, requiring good biodiversity, are an integral part of keeping the climate stable.

## ENERGY AND ECOSYSTEM HEALTH

Burning fossil fuels also is accelerating climate change. It has already wreaked havoc on many ecosystems, in some cases transforming entire landscapes and destroying biodiversity. We've been burning fossil fuels since the middle of the eighteenth century. These fuels, made of carbon from plants and animals that lived millions of years ago, have been stored in the Earth's crust where the right conditions caused that stored carbon to become oil, coal, and natural gas. When we burn fossil fuels, carbon that has been stored for millions of years is released into the atmosphere, throwing off the Earth's carbon balance and its ecosystem health. But the damage doesn't stop there. Getting the fuels out of the ground and processing and transporting them to their ultimate fiery use also has a tremendous ecological cost.

## Coal's Damage to Ecosystems

The United States currently gets slightly more than half of its electricity from coal. That amount is closer to three-quarters for many countries, including China, India, Australia, and Greece, whereas South Africa and Poland get practically all of their electricity from coal. Coal contains many impurities, such as sulfur and mercury, which are released into the atmosphere when the coal is burned. We have already discussed the effects of mercury on humans in the food chapter. It's likely, however, that mercury has similar effects on nonhuman animals, harming their nervous systems; jeopardizing their ability to hunt, forage, and raise their young; and diminishing their chances of survival.

Coal also ruins our air quality and produces the contaminant sulfur dioxide, a mild acid. Rains wash this acid onto plants and into the soils and waterways, harming the plants as well as aquatic wildlife and contributing to habitat loss and loss of biodiversity. The eastern half of the United States has been damaged the most from acid rain, with the states just south of the Great Lakes, the Northeast, and the Mid-Atlantic states bearing the brunt of the harm. Similar acid rain damage has occurred throughout the world.

Getting the coal out of the ground is perhaps most damaging to ecosystems. Throughout the central Appalachian Mountains, primarily in the states of West Virginia, Kentucky, and Virginia, coal companies are leveling the ancient mountains with a more cost-effective form of strip mining. *Mountain-top removal* uses dynamite to blast gargantuan amounts of earth off the top of the coal bed, which is then dumped into adjacent valleys. Not only does this destroy the forest ecosystem on the mountain tops—by conservative estimates, some 350 square miles of mountain land have been destroyed—but also more than 1,200 miles of valley stream ecosystems have been obliterated below.[12]

## Oil's Damage to Ecosystems

As Earth's petroleum sources become diminished and we look for ways to acquire more petroleum, nontraditional sources, such as oil sands and oil shale, look more economically appealing, especially as the price of oil skyrockets. The higher economic cost of the additional energy required to extract and process those nontraditional oils is offset by the higher price a barrel of oil can fetch. Unfortunately, getting oil from these sources exacts far greater ecological costs as well. The largest oil sands deposits are located in northwestern Alberta, Canada, and cover an area about the size of England. Unlike the liquid crude oil that comes from oil wells, oil sands contain a mixture of clay, sand, and bitumen, a heavy, tar-like fossil fuel. This requires that the oil sands be strip mined, obliterating the forest ecosystems that overlay the oil sands deposits. To extract the bitumen, it must be heated up, which is currently done by using natural gas. It is then separated from the sand and clay using large amounts of water. For every barrel of resulting crude oil, four to five times as much water is required to process it, and two tons of oil sands must be removed from the Earth.

To remove oil from shale rock, the most common practice is to strip mine the rock and take it to a processing plant where the shale is heated to liquefy the oil. Considering the added greenhouse gas emissions, loss of forest ecosystems, and additional use of water resources, oil sands and oil shale are indeed costly energy sources.

## REDUCING THE IMPACT OF FOSSIL FUELS ON THE CLIMATE AND ECOSYSTEMS

### Energy Efficiency

By far the easiest and generally least expensive way to reduce emissions from the burning of fossil fuels and the ecological impact of their extraction is to increase our energy efficiency. Vehicles, small and large appliances, electronic equipment, industrial processes, buildings—anything that uses energy can be made more efficient. Companies must take the steps to manufacture these efficient products, possibly with government mandates and public demand as motivators. Likewise, the power plants that generate energy, as well as the processes by which energy is transmitted, stored, and delivered, can all be made more efficient.

Accomplishing more with less energy benefits everyone by reducing greenhouse gas emissions; producing less pollution; and saving money for industry, businesses, and consumers. Fortunately, we already have the technology to make huge improvements in efficiency. What we lack is the political will to require it to happen. Individuals, organizations, and politicians themselves should push for reductions in greenhouse gas emissions through local, national, and international policies that encourage the transition to improved energy efficiency. They can use such incentives as tax credits, government programs to educate people about how to improve efficiency, mandates to industry to improve efficiency in consumer goods, and prices for goods and services that accurately reflect the amount of greenhouse gas emissions they produce.

A recent report by the American Solar Energy Society, which was reviewed by some of the country's top climate-change scientists, showed that we could make more than half of the 80 percent reduction in $CO_2$ emissions needed by 2050 by increasing energy efficiency. The remaining portion could be achieved by boosting renewable energy, which we'll talk about shortly.[13] Although additional research and development will be needed to maximize energy efficiency to the extent needed by 2050, current technologies are enough for us to begin making significant cuts in greenhouse gas emissions.

## Geoengineering

Geoengineering refers to direct and intentional human management of the climate system. Scientists have suggested several methods of managing the climate to slow or reverse global warming, including injecting sulfur dioxide into the atmosphere. Sulfur dioxide aerosols (acidic molecules in the air) have been released into our atmosphere for decades as an unwanted byproduct of burning coal for energy. These molecules are the source of acid rain, which has caused extensive damage to forests and waterways. In spite of this nasty result, sulfur dioxide is pretty effective at reflecting the Sun's energy back into space so that it doesn't warm Earth's surface. If these sulfur dioxide aerosols could be injected far enough up into the upper atmosphere, using balloons or guns, scientists suggest that they probably wouldn't cause more acid rain and could help slow global warming.

Another suggestion is to use mirrors to reflect sunlight back into space. This could be accomplished either by injecting small metallic particles into the upper atmosphere or by floating balloons with mirrors in the upper atmosphere. Still another option may be to mimic the reflective properties of snow and ice—which we're rapidly losing because of climate change— by covering parts of the ocean with white foam to reflect sunlight.[14, 15]

These various schemes may sound like science fiction, but scientists are worried enough about the state of our planet that they're seriously considering some form of geoengineering. The downside of all these schemes is that they really are science fiction—we've never tried deliberately managing the climate before, and we can only guess what the unintended consequences might be. Moreover, if such a strategy is used to forestall the warming process and we haven't drastically altered how we live to reduce our carbon emissions, we could be in even greater trouble. At some time in the future, if the "technofix" fails the accumulated carbon emissions could catapult our climate into a runaway global warming that would be cataclysmic in a very short time and would be virtually unstoppable. Another concern is that all of these schemes would be tremendously expensive. Opponents of geoengineering argue that the money would be more wisely spent making changes that will provide long-lasting, dependable protection against global warming and climate chaos.

Still another type of geoengineering "fix" focuses on altering what happens to the carbon we already emit. It involves capturing the carbon before it gets into the atmosphere and sequestering it somewhere on Earth to keep it out of the atmosphere. Possibilities for this kind of geoengineering include artificially making the oceans more alkaline (changing the pH) so that they can absorb more $CO_2$, which causes ocean water to become more acidic. Another suggestion is to "fertilize" the oceans with extra iron to allow plankton to absorb more $CO_2$. Again, the unintended consequences of these actions are unknown, and they could be grave.

In the chapter on air, we discussed the carbon capture and storage method proposed for coal-fired power plants. Briefly, this scheme involves capturing $CO_2$ before it leaves the smokestack and injecting it into the Earth's crust to store it and keep it out of the atmosphere. This technology is not yet feasible, and it could produce severe harm to the climate if the $CO_2$ were to accidentally leak out from the Earth's crust. Nevertheless, many experts and politicians are calling for new coal-fired power plants to be compatible with this technology so that it can be used as soon as the kinks are worked out.

## ALTERNATIVES TO FOSSIL FUELS

### Renewable Energy

To prevent climate change, the next best thing to improving energy efficiency is to get energy from clean, renewable sources that don't generate $CO_2$. Examples of renewable sources include energy from wind, the Sun, waves and currents, and tidal changes, to name a few.

Wind is one of the most common renewable energy sources, and the technology has already come a long way in the past few decades. Although windmills have been in use for centuries, their efficiency has increased by huge amounts recently. Advances in windmill design have drastically reduced these structures' harm to birds. They no longer provide roosting sites, for example, and the blades move slowly enough that birds can dodge them. Shutting down windmills during bird migrations has also saved bird lives. Of more concern currently is the number of bats that windmills have killed. Less is known about bat behavior, but scientists are working closely with the windmill industry to make windmills safer for bats, too. Of course, climate change and habitat destruction pose a far greater risk to both birds and bats than windmills do, but it's still important to reduce bird and bat fatalities.

Solar energy is another source of renewable energy that can be collected in a variety of ways. Photovoltaics, or "solar panels," can be installed on rooftops in most parts of the United States; they provide electricity directly into the existing electrical grid and could supply 10 percent of our energy needs by 2030. Rooftop solar hot-water heaters are much less expensive and pay for themselves in a few years.

Meanwhile, concentrated solar power installations require large expanses of treeless land and intense sunlight and use large, shiny metal surfaces to focus the sunlight on a central collecting point. The solar industry estimates that there is enough suitable land in California, Arizona, Nevada, and New Mexico to provide nearly seven times the amount of electricity currently used in the United States. Small concentrated solar power projects have already been installed in the U.S. Southwest. A larger project is being considered for the Sahara Desert that would provide electricity to northern Africa and Europe.[13]

In addition to wind and solar power, renewable energy can be generated from water currents in oceans and rivers and from changing tides. Projects to produce power from turbines placed in tidal basins are already in position at the mouth of the Hudson River in New York. The currents are so strong that the turbines have been damaged, but the power-generating potential is huge and companies are working out the problems. The marine ecosystem is being carefully monitored, and so far the fish seem to be quite capable of avoiding the moving turbine blades.

Hydroelectric power is sometimes included in the renewable energy category. Placing a small turbine into a river or creek is unlikely to cause significant damage to the ecosystem and can provide enough electricity for several houses or a small village. Damming up a large river, on the other hand, can provide much larger amounts of electricity, but it also does a lot of damage to the ecosystem upstream and downstream. More-over, the term *renewable* may not continue to apply. As climate change causes water to become scarcer in many areas, there may not be enough water flow to continue to produce electricity. With droughts and water shortages becoming more of a problem in many parts of the world, com-petition among farmers, cities, industry, and electricity generators could get much stiffer for the remaining water in rivers. In the United States, all the major rivers have already been dammed, so expanding large-scale hydroelectric power is not feasible. In fact, as a result of the damage to ecosystems that dams create, some dams are being dismantled. Small-scale hydroelectric power is still possible in many areas of the United States and has tremendous potential globally.

## Nuclear Energy

Nuclear power is a hot-button "alternative energy" issue. There's no doubt that once a nuclear power plant is built, it produces energy almost carbon-free for the life of the plant—usually four to five decades. The building of the plant, however, requires massive amounts of cement and other construction materials, and these materials release large amounts of carbon into the atmosphere as they are produced and transported to the plant site.

Maybe more of a problem, nuclear plants require uranium to make energy. Experts estimate there is only enough high-grade uranium in the Earth's crust to produce nuclear-generated energy for 60 to 70 years at current rates of generation. Once the high-grade ore has been used, much more energy will be required to process lower grades of ore, and that pro-cessing will produce carbon emissions. Also, when a nuclear plant reaches the end of its life, it must be carefully dismantled; that process also releases carbon. If the carbon released during construction, uranium processing, dismantling, and transportation of materials is all taken into account, the energy produced by nuclear power plants involves about the same amount of carbon emissions as wind-produced energy—and that's as long as high-grade uranium ore is available. Once the high-grade ore is gone, the carbon emissions increase to about the same amount as natural gas–fired power plants.[16] Aside from the issue of carbon emissions, nuclear power plants require even more water than coal-fired power plants; and, because the water is used for cooling, warm water won't do. This will be an increasingly difficult problem for nuclear power plants in a drought-stricken, warmer world. Solar and wind-generated electricity, on the other hand, require only minuscule amounts of water.

Of course, windmills don't create radioactive waste that will remain deadly for eons and must be transported to a repository—if one is eventually built—or stored on site. Windmills are also unlikely to be targeted by terrorists, and no one has to worry that materials found in windmills will be used to create weapons of mass destruction.

## A FINAL WORD ON ECOSYSTEMS

Before we describe some solutions to these myriad risks for ecosystem harm, we want to reiterate that climate change and other human-created forces—our fossil fuel consumption, land and water use, and over-fishing among them—join together to put at risk the planet that sustains us. Although we often consider climate change to be separate from those other forces, they are inextricably intertwined in a web of interactions that puts our health, and the health of our only planet, in peril. Given this reality, we simply have no choice but to seek solutions to these interconnected threats if we are to thrive.

## SOLUTIONS

We've already described many specific solutions to our ecosystem woes in previous chapters. Here we'll cover some of the other important individual and community solutions in which you can be engaged.

### Individual Solutions

- Reduce your pollution.
  - Never dump used oil from cars, other fossil fuels, pesticides, paints, solvents, or other household chemicals down drains or into sewers. They are lethal for aquatic ecosystems. Take them to toxic waste-collection sites for safe disposal. Better yet, don't use them in the first place—if you can avoid it.
  - Similarly, don't dispose of batteries—which are filled with toxins—or household chemicals in regular trash because they can leach out of landfills and into groundwater.
  - Don't burn your trash outside, even if you live in the country. The toxins released into the air will cause damage to plants, soil, and waterways.
- Reduce the amount of the resources that you use. Everything comes from somewhere, and its production, transport, use, and disposal invariably have an environmental impact.
- Reuse items as often as possible before disposal and recycle everything you can.

- Improve your energy efficiency and reduce your energy use.
- Help your family, neighbors, friends, and coworkers understand how important healthy ecosystems are to our health and well-being and how interconnected we really are.
- Get active in the political process. Let policy makers know that ecosystem issues are important to you. Vote accordingly.

## Community Solutions

- Produce more of your own energy, food, and other resources.
- Encourage biodiversity in backyards; in green spaces, such as parks and recreation areas; and in neighborhoods. The National Wildlife Federation has information about how to create backyard wildlife habitat. To learn more, visit http://www.nwf.org/backyard/.

## Regional, National, and International Solutions

- Work with governments and organizations to enact policies that mandate pollution reduction, resource-use reductions, and energy reductions.
- Support efforts to conserve biodiversity hotspots in developing countries by providing economic compensation to governments and local communities for not developing those regions. Forgiving some of their national debt in exchange for nature conservation is one mechanism. Reimbursing developing countries for income lost from not allowing resource extraction on sensitive lands is another. Research has shown that the more biodiversity a tropical forest has, the more carbon it stores.[17] These policies will help all of Earth's residents stabilize the climate.

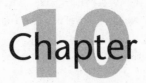

# Chapter 10

# Human Behavior:
# Choice to Change

Maria sits at her kitchen table, nervously tapping her finger on the wood surface, feeling the warmth pressing in around her. She stares out the window to the backyard that was once green but now is a drab brown. She waits for the doorbell to ring. Her kids are upstairs resting because the outdoor air quality is horrible today and they are both feeling unwell. Moravia is in the den, trying to get some work done even though it's the weekend, maybe avoiding what's coming. Max and his family are expected today.

As she stares at the bare patch of dirt outside where her prized flower bed once grew with abundance before the severe watering restrictions and the heat and the air pollution, Maria tries to think about what she could have done differently. And what could her community, her country, and the world have done to prevent the climate change that is reshaping everyone's lives, reshaping the planet, harming so many people, creatures, and plants?

Certainly, once the storms got much worse, the coasts became inundated, the water began to disappear, the heat persisted, and the crops grew strangely, then national and local politicians began to act. They passed laws to restrict energy use, increase taxes on consumption, and develop more renewable energy resources. Around the world nations enacted their own patchwork of policies to turn back global warming. But the efforts came slowly and long after scientists began to caution that time was of the essence, warning people to change their way of life or suffer dire consequences at the hands of a warming planet.

Maria thinks to herself, "Why didn't we actually do something about global warming before it was clear we were in big trouble, before it began to cause so much damage to the planet, before we all started suffering?" And then the ring of the doorbell startles Maria from her troubled thoughts.

## WHERE HUMAN BEHAVIOR AND CLIMATE CHANGE MEET

We are capable of creating monumental harm to ourselves: wars, nuclear holocaust, climate change. And we are capable of preventing our arrival at the brink of such destruction. If the researchers from myriad fields— psychology, sociology, political science, economics, communications, and more—were able to probe human behavior well enough to fully explain why humans create and can also undo such great harm, we might not have arrived at our latest precipice—climate chaos.

Many have tried and will keep trying to define why we can be so self-destructive and then, once we see the oncoming harm, often behave in a self-preserving fashion. This entire book has outlined how individual actions and the behavior of our institutions—government, corporate, business, academic, or other—have contributed to the force of climate change and its potential for ruinous harm to the health of living creatures around the globe. And then it has spelled out potential solutions to that harm.

Now, as this book comes to a close, it's time to seek an understanding of how our behavior has contributed to global warming and how we might be able to act differently to prevent its looming risks. We will not address such broad themes as world population, capitalism, and technological advances, which certainly involve human behavior and play vital roles in global warming and other environmental problems.[1] Although these topics are worthy of examination, they are beyond most of our abilities to influence. We will hope our society does find ways to limit their damage though—and quickly—by using some of the methods described in this book.

Moreover, because the research on the intersection between climate change and behavior is so new and limited, this chapter of necessity culls from related research on the environmental choices people make. And one pervasive generality from the research must be noted at the outset: Even as we've become more knowledgeable about climate change, and even though knowledge clearly is vital to our ecological behavior, there is still a big gap between our awareness of and intention to act in environmentally healthy ways and actually doing so.[2-4] This means that we know we need to do something about the harmful climate change we've played a role in creating, but more often than not we don't act on it. In the next few pages, we will look at what's at the heart of this discrepancy and what we can do about it.

Although we haven't the space to fully address the many variables that make human behavior so difficult to understand and to modify, this chapter nonetheless proposes that we have the potential to change to save ourselves from global warming before it becomes too detrimental to our well-being. Behavior change certainly explains how diverse people came together to defeat Nazism during World War II and how nuclear holocaust has so far failed to become a global reality. It also can explain how individuals, policy makers, power brokers, and social movements will begin to change their behavior, as outlined in all of this book's chapters, to save the planet from the life-threatening rising temperatures associated with climate change.

## HOW WE COME TO BEHAVE

If we're going to seek behavior change to fight global warming, it's instructive to briefly review how we have come to act as we do. Human development studies have found that our behavior is a function of some of the following mechanisms, which we've couched for this book's purposes in an environmental context:[5]

- We learn to behave through associations that are rewarded and punished, such as learning to turn off unnecessary lights or turn down the air conditioner or furnace so our utility bills cost less.
- We behave by making direct observations, such as seeing others recycling and doing so ourselves as a result.
- We choose to act through the process of resolving the differences between our beliefs and our behaviors. We may buy a more fuel-efficient vehicle to replace our beloved gas guzzler, for instance, because we learn that we need to reduce our $CO_2$ emissions and save on gas.
- We take into account costs and benefits as we make choices, such as deciding to pay a little more now to conserve energy to save the planet from climate change later. (You will soon see, though, that we're not so good at this.)
- And we are great at acting according to the social, cultural, and physical norms with which we live—including those stemming from our friends, spiritual or religious beliefs, education, and communities.

These are only a few of the most common ways in which we come to behave as we do. It's also essential to remember that human behavior, although malleable to some extent, is shaped to a great degree early in our lives. Children learn from their families, friends, teachers, the media, and the world around them, and it's not long before kids have formed habits that can affect them for the rest of their lives.[6] Habits, patterns of behavior that we engage in without thinking, hinder changing our behavior when we are faced with such risks as global warming.[7] Before we delve into this more, let's look at what behavior change might entail to understand what we're up against if we're going to act differently to prevent climate chaos.

## HOW WE CHANGE OUR BEHAVIOR

Knowing how we come to behave as we do is useful, but learning about how we can change our behavior is essential if we're to tackle climate change. Here are some of the most popular explanations for how we change our behavior when we are faced with a problem.

- We move through stages of behavior change, which begin with a lack of awareness of a problem, new awareness of the problem, a plan to deal with the problem, actual behavior that addresses the problem, evaluation of the outcome, and then maintenance of the new problem-solving behavior.[7]
- Others have tweaked that stage model, suggesting that conditions must be present for behavior change. These conditions include having anxiety about the need to change behavior, a willingness to take risks, support from others to change, and hope that changing won't be too difficult and will result in something positive.[8]
- Behavior change also may require that we set goals and make commitments to meet them and then have beliefs and a sense of ability to carry them out.[9,10]
- Some suggest that other elements must be in place to elicit behavior change, including concern, values, and a sense of personal responsibility.[11]
- And behavior change may depend on other factors, such as our receptiveness to innovation, responses to advertising campaigns, and, of course, reactions to policies and laws that require us to act differently.

Invariably, what's important here is to recognize that how we act and the ability to change our actions is amazingly complex and has no single driver. Underlying individual behavior are such complicated terms as personality, disposition, habits, attitudes, values, beliefs, and more, and the definitions of those terms aren't always precise. Moreover, although much of the research focuses on individual factors, it's becoming increasingly clear in environmental studies that human behavior change truly resides at the intersection of individuals and their communities.[12] If we are to deter the risks of climate chaos, behavior change must happen not only because of who we are inside and what we do but in the way we and the world around us interrelate. Before getting to that crossroads, let's explore where most of the research about environmental behavior has taken place—with individuals.

## INDIVIDUALS AND CLIMATE CHANGE

### Brains and Behavior

A lot goes on in the individual brain to elicit behavior, which accounts for the number of variables researchers are studying to determine whether humans might be ecological, or pro-environmental, when faced with such problems as climate change. Some of those variables include:[13,14]

- factual knowledge about the environment
- concerns, attitudes, and beliefs about the environment and ecological behavior
- social and moral values and norms regarding the environment
- the intention to behave in ecologically sound ways
- a sense of responsibility for and ability to behave ecologically
- a variety of so-called moderators, which include gender, race, socioeconomic status, group membership, political affiliation, educational level, and nationality

Because climate change has only become big news in recent years, the way these variables influence our behavior toward climate change isn't always clear. The research is more certain about two pronounced ways that people approach the natural environment.[15,16] On the one hand, it appears that many people have an underlying value that Earth and its resources are there for the taking to make human lives better through economic development. On the other, some people have the value that Earth and its resources must be husbanded if people are to exist in harmony with the world around them and flourish. Although these values are not mutually exclusive, these two ways of perceiving the world are essential to keep in mind as we pursue the connection between our behavior and climate change.

Add to this that most U.S. citizens, and many people around the world, believe:[9,17]

- they are environmentalists
- that climate change is happening and it will cause significant harm
- that they'd be willing to pay something to prevent climate change

Yet many of us don't do much when we are presented with the need to address our individual behavior and the community and institutional policies that are causing climate change and other environmental problems.[18] If it's going to compromise our lifestyles much, we balk.

Remember when we talked about the gap between what individuals say and do about the environment? This discrepancy between beliefs and behaviors toward climate change has varied and tenacious roots:[12,19–21]

- Climate change is too difficult a concept to fully understand, so although we believe it exists we don't know what it really means.
- We feel individually powerless to do anything about climate change.
- We believe only politicians and corporations have the power to address global warming.[9]
- We fear climate change and its costs to our taxes, lifestyles, and comfortable habits, so we deny that it's really that bad.
- Alternatively, some people tend to think positively about climate change and believe events are more controllable than not, minimizing the need for action.
- The effects of global warming also aren't particularly evident now or locally. They are more apt to be a problem elsewhere later—so why act now?
- When the effects do occur, say through more-powerful storms or rising sea levels, it's not clear that climate change is the direct cause . . . and the harmful outcomes usually seem to abate.
- We think in the short term, so any given *cool* day dissipates our concern about global *warming*.
- We appear to feel more responsibility to act on local environmental problems than on global ones, even if we believe global environmental problems are more serious than our local ones.[22]
- Many of us believe we will come up with technological fixes for climate change anyway, so there's no need to worry now.
- Because most other people aren't responding much, it seems that our immediate action is not needed.
- Some people are simply apathetic about the issue.
- Other people might be concerned about the climate, but they believe that capitalism and free markets need to function without impediments.[23]
- Finally, for many there are more important issues, such as the economy, homeland security, education, health care, housing, poverty, and more.

   The first bullet in that long list of reasons for not acting to deter climate change deserves a bit more commentary before we move on: Although most of us believe climate change is real and potentially dangerous, we also believe that reducing the emissions that cause it can be delayed until there is even more evidence it's going to be truly harmful.[17] Importantly, this doesn't involve just downplaying the seriousness of climate change. We may be complacent because our brains don't grasp that climate-harming $CO_2$ emissions going into the atmosphere far exceed those that are being removed from the atmosphere. Reducing new emissions, therefore, requires enormous effort immediately if we are to stave off the cascading harm that those emissions will bring to climate change.

   There is an additional reason to question our behavior toward global warming. Research indicates that our minds use automatic mechanisms to simplify the overabundance of information in the world around us. Brains on autopilot allow bad habits to flourish and may stop us from taking action on problems that may turn out to be irreversible if we don't act quickly. Let's take a look at some of these mechanisms so central to our ecological behavior:[5,6,24]

- *Discounting.* A term often used in economics, discounting means we give less value to the future—we discount it—in favor of our current lives.[25] Discounting allows us to go on consuming fossil fuels to live as well as we can now even if that means more global warming and harm to public health in the future.[11]
- *Peak experiences.* We are more interested in immediate, feel-good experiences than in long-term average trends. We focus on what's right before us, not what's ahead. Thus, we will engage in activities that may deepen global warming without thinking of the harm those activities will cause through time.
- *Optimism bias.* Some people are more optimistic or refuse to accept anything but a positive spin on a difficult situation.[26,27] Add peak experiences and discounting to optimism bias and it's difficult to see the realities of climate change.
- *Losses versus Gains.* We tend to feel losses more than gains, and we also tend to want to avoid an immediate loss at all costs even if such a loss might result in a long-term gain. In regard to global warming, we perceive measures that restrict our climate-changing behavior as painful and avoid them. Or we avoid changing our own behavior because it might make us feel as if we've lost something.
- *Confirmation bias.* People evaluate new information in a selective, or biased, manner to confirm already existing beliefs. If we don't believe that climate

change is happening, we pay more attention to the naysayers who support our views.

- *Single-action bias.* People are likely to engage in one action to reduce a perceived risk and believe that no more action is needed to reduce the risk.[11] We might, for example, purchase a hybrid car as our one way of addressing global warming but continue to live in an enormous, energy-inefficient home without a second thought.
- *Availability* and *simulation.* Events that easily come to mind and are easier to imagine, or simulate, may seem to be more likely to happen.[28] This can make it difficult for people to envision climate change and to act to avoid its repercussions because they haven't experienced them personally or they can't imagine them.
- *Scarcity.* People tend to value what is scarce or seems to be running out. This could be a good or a bad thing. On the good side, if people perceive that climate change is making clean air, water, food, and other essentials more scarce, we might value them more and change our behavior to protect them. But we might also begin to hoard these scarce resources, which could create more conflicts.
- *Denial.* Good old denial. Most of us know this term, which refers to refusing to see what's facing us to protect the comforts we associate with the status quo.[29-31]

The point of this list of automatic mental mechanisms that hinder our ability to deal with climate change—and there are more—is to repeat this amazing thing about the human mind: Even when we are presented with accurate information about the harm that climate change will cause, research shows that time and again we will use automatic processes that prevent us from addressing the threat. So we develop patterns of behavior, many of them habitual, and then cling to them through mental means that keep us from recognizing just how risky those habits are in the face of global warming. This is one reason that education alone doesn't help us change our behavior. We must dig deeper into individual characteristics to find some hope that we can rise to the challenge that climate change is presenting us.

## Environmental Concern and Emotions

With the growing volume of talk about climate change in the media, education, and general discourse, it should be no surprise that many polls and studies show the number of people who are concerned about global warming has been rising. In recent years, more than half—and sometimes three-fourths or more—of the populations studied say they are concerned.[32] How concern affects behavior, it turns out, is one of the most-studied concepts in environmental research.

You might think that increased concern about climate change or other environmental problems, whether they're risks to favorite creatures and places or harm to oneself, would be reason enough to actually do something to care for the environment. Early research wasn't so positive. Many studies found that people with stronger concerns weren't necessarily more prone to act on them than people who had weaker concerns.[11,33] Part of the problem was the difficulty assessing concern and behavior, but the gap between what goes on in our brains and what we do is also present in the relationship between environmental concern and ecological action.

More recent studies do suggest that we are more likely to behave in ecological ways—for example, recycling, using public transportation, or buying organic food—when we have stronger concerns about the environment.[34] Other factors, such as an awareness of what to do, ease in acting, and low cost to act, add to this response. This suggests a possible countercurrent to our automatic mind mechanisms.

But it's not all good: Studies often find that people in the United States have less concern about the environment than people from other nations.[16,35,36] Moreover, although a higher proportion of people in wealthier nations favor environmental protection over economic growth, people in poorer countries often express more concern for taking care of their local environment than people in wealthier nations. That is true even if those wealthier nations have more resources to attend to environmental quality.[37,38] This may be because poorer people are more aware of their dependence on nature than their more well-to-do peers in industrialized lands.

If we look at what influences concern about climate change, our beliefs and attitudes appear to be among the most important factors.[39] We'll talk more about those factors in the next section. Imposing on them are these elements:

- messages about climate change along with their trustworthiness
- personal experience of global warming
- knowledge and thinking about climate change
- evaluations and consequences of the issue
- our sense of personal responsibility for global warming
- our hope that policies will effectively address climate change

At its most basic, those factors combine to influence how concerned we are about climate change. People who have the strongest beliefs, most negative attitudes, and greatest certainty about global warming and its consequences are more likely to support government efforts to enact policies that reduce air pollution as one cause of climate change. But if you don't feel overly responsible for the problem, believe you can't do much about it, or are simply afraid of the issue because of the news reports you hear about it, those factors may reduce your concern and your effort to do anything about climate change.[20,29,40]

How we talk to ourselves about our environmental concern also can lead to inaction. For one thing, we tend to envision energy as being readily replaceable and used for life's necessities rather than being wasted; therefore, people can ignore the reality of "waste" that is central to conservation practices.[41] In addition, we persistently compare our levels of concern to others' levels, and in so doing we tend to perceive ourselves as users of natural resources but others as wasters of those resources. These almost automatic processes allow individuals to justify how they behave toward the environment: We blame others for resource consumption that fuels climate change, or we perceive that resources are renewable to justify our consumption of those resources. .

One of the important, if obvious, implications about concern is that if we could get more people to be truly concerned about global warming, we might reach a tipping point of human action to prevent it. We have to be careful, though, about how we influence people to be concerned. It appears that persuading people to be more concerned about climate change works best if the focus is on how it will harm them directly, say through reduced food production or damage to their homes.[39] It's not as important to focus on how local creatures or scenery will be harmed. The subtle difference here is that we are more concerned and more involved when we can attach the relevance of climate change's harm to resources vital for our own existence.

All of this talk about concern leads us here: Part of what underlies our concern about climate change is how we feel about it. Although there isn't much research on emotions as they relate to global warming, except for fear, which we'll discuss shortly, several studies indicate our emotional connection with nature motivates us to want to protect it.[42,43] It's also evident that our feelings about climate change may motivate us to seek its resolution.[32,44,45] But if we feel too uncomfortable, we may come to deny the seriousness of the climate problem so we end up not being as concerned.[46]

Even though environmental concern has been extensively studied, it turns out this concern is not a great predictor of our behavior toward the environment, such as reducing energy consumption to stave off climate change.[47,48] Other factors, such as how we think—with our attendant attitudes, beliefs, and values—also play a role.

## Thinking: Beyond Concern to Attitudes, Beliefs, Values. . . .

Thinking about climate change may work with our concern to counter the automatic mental processes that result in inaction to deter global warming's harm. Some research does suggest this, but it's complicated.

At its most basic level, thinking evolves from our attitudes and beliefs, which stem from our underlying values, or the rules that guide our choices.[48-50] One of the simplest ways to distinguish our environmental values is by breaking them down into self-centered, people-centered, and nature-centered values.

- Climate change's harm needs to be reduced because it's going to hurt *me*.
- Climate change's harm needs to be reduced because it's going to hurt lots of *people*.
- Climate change's harm needs to be reduced because it's going to hurt *nature*.

In all three cases, which need not be mutually exclusive, strong values to address climate change may exist. As noted already, another common values distinction is that some of us believe humans are part and parcel of nature and need to nurture it, whereas others believe we are separate from nature and can use its resources as we need them to benefit humanity.

It's all well and good to understand that our values inform our attitudes and beliefs and, thereby, our thinking. That suggests that we might want to alter our values and how they contribute to our thinking so we could think in ways that would truly attend to climate change. But changing your values, often imparted from the family and world in which you develop, isn't an easy process. And, like concern, there may be a gap between our values and how we act on them.[18]

It appears we might be able to narrow the gap somewhat if we look at the strongest associations between brain and behavior:[3,51-53]

- Our knowledge of, beliefs about, and values toward the environment are important precursors to intending to behave in ecological ways, and that intention predicts actually behaving ecologically.
- Although generally positive attitudes and values toward the environment enhance a willingness to care for it, when we have knowledge about specific

ecological actions, how to carry them out, and a sense that we can succeed at them, we're even more likely to do so.

- Additive elements, including feelings of guilt, social norms, specific implementation plans, and a moral stance, appear to improve our intentions to engage in ecological behavior.[13,14,54]

So, it's good to have environmental knowledge and values and know specific things you can do to act on those values, but the motivation to do them and other internal and external pressures—perhaps economic or political pressures—are vital to behaving in ecological ways. If we take the time to think about the consequences of an ecological behavior, think about what will make it easy or difficult to carry out that behavior, and think about the social setting in which such behavior will be carried out, we're more likely to do so.

Now here's where it gets even more interesting. It turns out that thinking and environmental concern may work in concert. People who have stronger environmental concern appear to have more situation-specific thinking about how difficult it will be to carry out an environmentally responsible behavior, and if they have higher levels of concern they may work harder to overcome those barriers.[47] Meanwhile, people who have less environmental concern think more about acting in responsible ways primarily if the social setting suggests it. This means that people who aren't too environmentally concerned may still benefit from social support to behave ecologically.

You can see that your intention to protect the planet from climate change is moderated by your level of environmental concern; your thinking (with all of your attendant values, attitudes, and beliefs) about the specific behaviors you can engage in; and the possible outcomes, barriers, and social support you face in behaving to save the planet. Acting to address global warming isn't as simple as just having concern or being able to think about climate change and its repercussions.

In this discussion about how values underpin our beliefs, attitudes, thinking, and concern to influence our behavior, it's easy to ignore an important problem: If our value system supports economic development at all costs to improve people's lot; concerns itself with immediate self-gratification through the extensive use of nature's apparently endless bounty; or has faith in technological, political, or institutional solutions to any problem, then whatever information we encounter about climate change will end up twisted to support our values, possibly resulting in inaction or paralysis.[18,55] It turns out that people who have these common values are less concerned about environmental problems and the need to do something to solve them.

Of course, we've established that many of us have strong beliefs about the need to be ecologically sound, but we are likely to think this way as long as our current social, political, and economic processes are not changed by it.[56] In this manner, we can be pro-environment but unwilling to pay extra taxes, alter the traditional economy, or otherwise upend the existing status quo that is contributing to climate change. This suggests that social, political, and economic beliefs are more pervasive than beliefs about the environment, which is not too surprising given that our concern about such environmental issues as climate change hasn't been around as long as those other beliefs.

There is an alternative, to be sure. We can value and think about the interconnectedness of people and the planet. We can see that the Earth has scarce resources that need to be carefully tended to preserve life. We can change the way we behave through structuring our lives, our economy, and our political processes to thrive without the need for endless consumption and growth—the main reasons for climate change—being our driving force.

Maybe we can overcome the discrepancy between our thinking and its relationship to our behavior—remember that gap—if we become more conscious about how our brains and behavior are contributing to climate change and seek alternatives to prevent it.[14,18] But, as we've noted, there are other factors at play in this relationship. Our perceptions of our communities' values, our levels of fear, and our sense of how much control we have to carry out our behavior also play roles in predicting our intentions to engage in environmental actions, such as recycling and composting.[11,57,58]

And then there's ambivalence, which is not knowing quite what you think about such issues as climate change. Research shows that people who are more ambivalent have less intention to behave in ecological ways.[59] Scientific uncertainty can fuel this ambivalence by allowing us to doubt the seriousness of a threat such as climate change.[60] Finding ways to attend to our ambivalence about climate change would seem prudent if we are to turn the tide against it. One way may be instilling a sense of responsibility toward and a belief in our ability to fend off global warming.

## Personal Responsibility and Self-Efficacy

People who have a strong sense of responsibility for problems such as climate change are more likely to engage in behaviors to resolve those problems.[40,61] That action may be heightened if they are part of and also feel responsible for a group that climate change could harm.

Responsibility also is linked to some of the other topics we've discussed so far. Those of us who feel responsible for resolving climate change benefit from gaining knowledge about the seriousness of the problem and, in turn, become more supportive of policies that could prevent it.[39] Moreover, those of us who see individual behavior and corporate industrial production, rather than natural processes, as responsible for climate change tend to believe that people should take responsibility for action to control it.[62]

Although many of us seem to be aware that we need to take responsibility for environmental problems, we may have trouble doing so because we see so few others acting responsibly.[2] Or, as previously noted, we may have difficulty acting if we feel more responsibility for local environmental problems than distant ones, even if we perceive the distant environmental problems as being more serious than the local ones.[63]

Linked to personal responsibility is a concept known as *self-efficacy*, or the perceived ability to engage in activities to address a problem or carry out an action. It's one thing to feel responsible to act and another to believe you can actually do it. Research indicates that people who believe their actions will make a difference and can carry them out are more likely to act than those who don't believe in their self-efficacy.[64] Self-efficacy may also explain why making goals and commitments to behave ecologically is an effective way to promote that behavior.[10]

In one study, self-efficacy was the primary factor behind the intention to deter climate change.[23] Self-efficacy and environmental knowledge appear to combine, moreover, to indicate a greater likelihood of individual political involvement or other action toward environmental problems, including climate change.[64,65] It also helps when the problems have clearly apparent causes that we can address, which is difficult when it comes to global warming.

Here's another connection between self-efficacy and personal responsibility. When people feel a responsibility to behave ecologically, it fuels their belief in their ability to do so, especially when they know the outcome will be positive.[66] The self-efficacy of some people, however, appears to be limited by the perception that acting alone in the face of environmental problems like climate change is fairly meaningless.[2] This hearkens back to having a social setting in which collective action stimulates individual behavior—the more others are doing, the more individuals are encouraged to take action, too.

There are some obvious barriers to self-efficacy and personal responsibility about climate change. Some people are lazy, unable to muster the fortitude to act, or believe the problem is beyond them. Others may believe that government and big business should shoulder the burden for addressing global warming or that technology will save the environment, which may diminish their individual sense of responsibility and ability to take action. Whatever our reasons for avoiding or taking responsibility for climate change and doing something about it, how much import we give the issue is based not only on our thinking and concern but also on how much risk we see in it. Risk and the fear it can engender, as we shall see, can be important behavioral motivators.

## Risk Perception and Fear

We've already established that most of us have concern that global warming is a real problem, but our perceptions about its risks for us and our levels of fear concerning those risks appear to play important roles in how we behave toward the threat it poses.[24,53,67-69] In general, greater perceptions of the risks from climate change, including awareness of the health impacts, appear to motivate more interest in doing something to prevent the risks and paying more to have them addressed—but not always.[45] Also, it appears people's beliefs about their ability to adapt to the risks of climate change can affect their perceptions about global warming and their behavior toward it.[70] If you think you'll be able to adapt, the risks may seem diminished. (As an aside, adaptation to some of global warming's harm may be possible and necessary; but if extreme events ensue, it's difficult to predict the outcomes for our health, much less the planet's![71-73])

Although individual differences influence our varied perceptions of risk, and although many of us may sense risks primarily when we hear about them in the media or other sources, mostly it appears that Americans perceive climate change as a moderate risk to people and the planet.[32,74] This seems to be the case when comparing risk perceptions of the lay public and risk professionals, with laypeople seeing climate change as a moderate risk and risk professionals putting it near the top of environmental risks. In addition, Americans also perceive that climate change is more likely to affect people and environments far away and in the distant future. People in other countries, such as Germany and Great Britain, also perceive that climate change presents some risk, mostly to others elsewhere later. So, many of us believe we'll have a good chance of adapting.

What's most paradoxical about this is that public opinion polls show we have strong media-driven concerns about climate change, but we don't make dealing with it a priority because we see the risks as only moderate and believe the harm is going to happen to others in places far away at some time in the future. Moreover, we have difficulty paying to reduce the potential harm of climate change because we discount the future and perceive economic investment as too great a loss in the present for a questionable benefit in the future. And there's an additional problem. Few people make the vital link between climate change and human health, even though that harm is likely to be one of the greatest threats global warming creates for humanity.[75] This book seeks to counter just that worrisome disconnection.

Worry is a central theme throughout this book, too. Although how much we worry is partly based on our levels of perceived danger from climate change as its effects unfold, we've said it repeatedly: There is ample data to show that climate change has the potential to devastate the health and well-being of millions of people on Earth—including you—as well as millions of other species and landscapes as we know them. If that isn't scary. . . . It turns out, though, that being fearful doesn't necessarily translate into motivation to change our behavior.[11,58] Fear also can inhibit action. Let's explain how this works.

First, we need a risk. For us, it's climate change, which we hear about in all sorts of messages from the media, people at work, and in educational settings. Second, those messages also communicate how severe and close to us the risk is, how susceptible we might be to it, and whether there's anything we can do about it (there's self-efficacy again!). Now, each of us, with our individual characteristics, takes those message components and does one of the following:

- We don't take action if we fail to believe the fear-arousing messages and thus classify the risk at a low level. In this case, we may not feel much, if any, fear and can easily ignore the message.
- We don't take action even though we believe the messages put the risk at a high level because we feel we can do little or nothing about the problem. Here we may feel a sense of hopelessness or paralysis to act. This is akin to learned helplessness, which describes the process by which we learn that there is seemingly nothing we can do about a problem and therefore give up trying. Or we may deny the threat and go so far as to reject its evident risks, leading to another sort of inaction.
- Finally, we are likely to take action when the messages say the risk is high and we have a sense that we can do something about it. This is where fear can motivate action.

Some recent research indicates that the unpleasant emotions we feel about global warming do allow us to avoid engagement in addressing the problem.[30] When we feel fear and related emotions about climate change, including helplessness and guilt, we may try to get them under control by distancing ourselves from the issue and not participating in activities to deter its harm.

On the other hand, emotions may motivate some people to act. Guilt might promote feelings of responsibility to the environment.[76] And people who are more worried about climate change lowering their living standards, engendering disease, and limiting food supplies report a greater willingness to make sacrifices to fight climate change than those who aren't so worried about those potential personal outcomes.[77] Fear also can help people have more positive attitudes toward energy-saving conservation measures.[78,79]

Interestingly, self-efficacy may give fear a boost to motivate behavior. It appears that when people have fear about a risk and a sense of self-efficacy to do something about that risk, that's a better predictor of resulting behavior to deal with the risk than when the fear stands alone.[58] It's evident that when media or other messages convey a high risk of climate change harming us where we live *and* give us some suggestions to deter those risks and the fear they engender in us, we're more likely to take action. More about the media's role in risk messages will be discussed later in the chapter.

Now, before we make it seem as if risk perception and fear can explain a lot of environmental behavior, we must add some complexity. First, we need to restate that unless environmental risks are immediate threats to people's sense of well-being, they may worry more about distant environmental risks even though they have less motivation to act on them because of their perceived distance.[11,80] So people likely would take action to limit pollution near their homes even if it's not much of a threat before they'd take action to prevent climate change's harm, which we know will be worse for humanity but seems to be a far-off prospect. Add to this that people consider how much control they have in doing anything about a risk, and you begin to see that those of us who worry more about a seemingly distant risk like climate change but believe we have little individual control to do anything about it might slip into learned helplessness.

Additionally in the realm of risks, recall how we discount the future and focus on preventing immediate losses to live a peak life now. Although some of us might say it's good to reduce the consumption in our current lifestyles if reducing our $CO_2$ emissions will prevent future climate change harm, others will argue that given the nebulous nature of distant global warming risks we might as well continue to live our current lifestyles.[11]

Let's address another complexity we discussed earlier. Optimistic thinking, which runs counter to fear, is the tendency some people have to think positively regardless of the risks we face; therefore, they fail to act on the risks.[40] Even optimistic people, however, will be more likely to engage in pro-environmental behavior if they perceive more risk, among other variables, from environmental problems.[27] And overly fearful people who make everything into a catastrophe—just the opposite of optimists—can fall into inaction through a sense of futility.

Clearly, using risk perception and fear to motivate people to change their behavior toward climate change isn't as simple as getting them to better understand the harm global warming portends. Although there is some evidence that people who have a more accurate understanding of the causes of climate change report a greater likelihood of acting to prevent it, recent examination of risk perception about climate change has found that simply giving people more accurate and detailed information doesn't necessarily translate into more behavior to fight those risks.[74,77] And then there's the problem that how we feel—rather than think—about climate change risks may deter us from action.[11,46] Moreover, many of us are willing to take action but only if it's easy to do so, doesn't cost too much, provides personal benefits, and involves honest government responses to the problem.[74,81] Ultimately, it's evident that many of us pay attention to climate change's risks and the fear they can generate, but a variety of processes hinder our efforts to prevent oncoming harm.[82] Some of these processes also are connected with our own characteristics, and this is the topic of the next section.

## Sociodemographic Variables

Each of us has certain characteristics, including gender, income, and education, and studies show that these characteristics can affect our ecological behavior. Before we touch on some of the most interesting characteristics, called sociodemographic variables, it's essential to recognize that lumping people together means making broad generalizations. Some of these variables, such as age and race, are inflexible. Others, such as education and income, can be influenced. Still, if we're to tackle global warming, it's instructive to know that some people are more likely than others to have specific thoughts, feelings, and behaviors toward this problem.

First, women tend to take environmental issues such as climate change more seriously than men and want to do something about it, even if they don't always actually do so.[87] There are some caveats, however, to this finding.[53,83]

Second, younger people, who are more educated and less concerned with environmental regulations, appear to be more willing to act to deter climate change but not necessarily to vote for more government interventions.[36,77] Younger people also are more willing to pay higher fuel prices to address environmental problems such as global warming.[84]

Third, regardless of age, people who are highly educated are more apt to believe in climate change and to support government programs to fight it.[39,85] But this doesn't necessarily hold up across nations.

Fourth, although we've already noted that people in poorer nations often are more concerned about the environment than people in wealthier nations, when researchers compare people in specific countries often the wealthier people report more concern about the environment than the less well-to-do.[48,86] Even so, one study found poorer people reported greater interest in doing the things necessary to reduce climate-changing emissions, whereas wealthier people were less willing to cut back on such behaviors as driving and home energy use.[77]

Fifth, when considering groups of people with similar characteristics, one study found that industry and government employees may perceive climate change as less of a risk than members of environmental groups and university researchers.[87]

You can see that gender, age, education, nationality, income, and group affiliation may be related to climate-change behavior. Other human characteristics, including race,[88–90] religion,[91–93] and political stance,[94,95] have been examined as they relate to environmental issues such as climate change with varied findings.

We also can look at broader patterns to better understand human behavior toward global warming. One study, for instance, found that people who forcefully debunk climate change as a myth are predominantly male, white, politically conservative, individualistic, and highly religious.[32] Although they make up less than 10 percent of the U.S. population, they are outspoken and well represented both in government and in big business. By contrast, people who say climate change is going to harm everything and everyone are more politically liberal, support government action to fight global warming, and are more likely themselves to have taken climate change action. According to this research, the latter group makes up slightly more than 10 percent of the U.S. population, although most other people in the study have views that are closer to these so-called "alarmists" than to the aforementioned "naysayers."

Figuring out how to work with these sociodemographic variables to improve behavior toward climate change isn't simple. It's difficult to persuade people to change their political beliefs, for example, and it's not easy to enhance education and income in any society, which seem to lead people to take action against global warming. In addition, there's little sense in using these variables to create more polarities among people, which only contribute to conflicts that hinder action. Still, we need to know about how these variables influence behavior and then understand how that behavior relates to the risk of global warming if we are to have hope for preventing its harm.

## Hope for Individual Behavior

Individual factors certainly are only part of the equation in preventing the peril that climate change presents. We will attend to some of the community factors in a moment. It's essential that we say now, though, that there is hope for us as individuals. Despite the gap between our growing knowledge of global warming and our behavior toward it, humans have demonstrated time and again that as risks rise we can rise together—with all of our individual differences—to the occasion to deter them. Although you may not believe that you as an individual can do much to alter the course of climate change, when individuals work with other people and the institutions that people have created, the potential to wage war against oppressors, deter sickness and death from natural and human-made maladies, and create a world that nurtures rather than destroys all are within human abilities. Let's now explore some of the factors in our communities that can help us in our struggle to prevent climate chaos.

## COMMUNITY FACTORS AND CLIMATE CHANGE

We don't behave exactly as we choose. The government entities that represent us, our local communities, our workplaces and schools, and even the corporations that manufacture what we buy affect our lives through their laws, policies, and products. At the outset of this chapter, we noted that individual characteristics combine with community or situational factors to result in the vast array of human behavior, and when people want to care for the environment they are most likely to do so when they perceive that community factors are in place to facilitate it.[57] People who have negative attitudes about ecological behavior and also perceive that community factors make it difficult to have an impact are the most likely not to act.

All of the research that shows a disconnection between people's individual characteristics and their environmental behavior points us in this new direction—community factors. Perhaps the gap between personal motivation and taking action toward climate change can be narrowed much more with the assistance of community factors pointing us in the right direction.

These community factors can run the gamut.[14,32,57] They can be government regulations and laws, such as mandates for fuel-efficient vehicles, homes, and businesses; absolute prohibitions on climate-damaging technologies; or various forms of economic incentives, subsidies, or taxes to encourage climate-protective efforts and discourage harmful behavior. They can be corporate and business initiatives to manufacture and sell products that don't harm the climate. They can be educational endeavors, advertising, or other forms of communication. They can even be more indistinct forces, such as the social groups to which we belong, the cultures in which we develop, and the places in which we live. Of course, all of these community factors may actually contribute an enormous share to environmental harm, but we have created them and we can change them, too.[12]

This section intends to briefly describe some of the community factors that play roles in our behavior toward climate change. Because there is less research on community factors—in part because it's much more difficult to examine the functioning of big structures than of individual people[96]—we begin with a limited look at economics. Money, to be sure, plays an enormous role in how we care about our planet and climate change.

## Economics

Let's be frank, many of us have faith in economic development to solve our problems.[20,97] Yet current economic models state that growth will mean more $CO_2$ emissions to fuel that growth, which only increases the rate of life-harming climate change.

Knowing the risk of unbridled economic growth while also having an appreciation for the value of our natural environment so we want to preserve it as a result, we enter into cost-benefit analyses:[22] This is the common practice of determining whether the cost of an item is tolerable considering how much we'll get out of it. If it costs little or nothing to reduce environment-damaging $CO_2$ emissions and we have easy accessibility to the means to do so, many of us would be doing it.[2] The trouble is, taking action that might hurt the economy, our jobs, and our current lifestyles (including our precious vehicles[98,99]) is hard for us to accept. Yes, we're willing to voluntarily take low-cost actions, such as purchasing energy-efficient light bulbs and appliances, but we're not up to more expensive and difficult actions, such as installing solar panels on our homes.[2,77] Also, we'd rather have incentives, rewards, and supportive feedback to do the right thing for the environment than face law-induced controls, such as consumption taxes or restrictions on our behavior, although even these inducements may not help our ecological behavior last long.[100,101] As governments, corporations, utility companies, and other organizations use similar cost-benefit analyses in their operations, you can see that economics presents a substantial barrier to addressing climate change.

Importantly, we seem to misunderstand that failing to pay now to reduce $CO_2$ emissions—often through greater efficiencies and increased taxes on those emissions—will cost us much more in the future, not only because of the incredibly expensive damage climate change will cause but also because we may have even fewer future resources to deal with the damage.[40] Moreover, it's really quite difficult to grasp the costs of climate change because they come in so many forms and with so many possible outcomes.[102] We can estimate economic, human, infrastructure, ecosystem, political, moral, and other costs, and we can do so for individuals or groups of various sizes on local, regional, national, and global levels. You can see how this might create confusion and make it difficult to assign monetary as well as social costs that would motivate us to act now.

Of course, we have to add to these difficult cost considerations our automatic brain processes, including discounting, peak experiences, and avoidance of losses. We certainly discount the future economic costs of climate change, which may seem incalculable if such change will damage and destroy millions of people's lives, homes, and livelihoods, so we focus instead on immediate financial costs and benefits. Even at that, the immediate costs to address climate change may seem too high to us; we'd rather not spend a lot today and continue to live as well as we do without "paying" much heed to the future.

Moreover, many of us perceive that the economic interests in government and corporations have much more financial power than the people, and in this way individual action toward climate change becomes minimized.[31] This may suggest that governments and corporations will need to set the economic tone for human behavior to prevent climate change. The next section addresses this topic.

## Government and Institutional Policies

As we've stated, governments, corporations, and other organizations clearly provide guidance for human behavior. Their laws and regulations;

various economic taxes, incentives, and subsidies; and wide array of products, promotions, and packaging play essential roles in our work, resource consumption, driving habits, schooling, and more.

Governments have long used laws, punishments, incentives, and other means to dictate our behavior.[5] If a business produces less $CO_2$, for example, that behavior might warrant a tax break. If it produces too much, there will be a fine. Such conditions have motivated other public health behavior, including the wearing of seat belts and the decline in tobacco use in recent decades. These conditions can promote personal responsibility, and they may impart a sense of self-efficacy, too.

Apart from the ability to set conditions, many of us look to government, businesses, and other institutions to be leaders in environmental matters because they have more economic and political power to effect change, even if we don't entirely trust them to do so.[31,103] If we perceive that people in power are being fair in their influence, we give them more authority to carry it out.[104]

Some researchers also argue that government, corporations, and local organizations should be at the forefront of shaping our climate-change prevention behavior by behaving themselves in ways that encourage it.[12,105] Because these institutions are creating some of the greatest environmental harm, it seems reasonable that they should shoulder more of the burden to reduce it.[106]

Others suggest that because people agree with government policies that don't affect them but disagree with policies that restrict their current way of living, governments and organizations should work harder to instill personal responsibility in their citizens that reduces the need for policies to ensure that people are doing the right thing.[5,32] To do so might require public education campaigns, incentives, and the decentralization of power to local communities.

When national governments fail to lead on preventing climate change, state and local governments may need to step up as the leaders.[107] One study found that municipal governments vary widely in their adoption of climate-protection policies. Among the reasons for greater local-government involvement in climate-change policies are closeness to other cities that have already enacted those policies; change agents and environmental activists who target them to adopt policies; connections with broader efforts on climate change; and an understanding of how the climate is linked to many other environmental concerns that affect communities.[108]

Yet, the trustworthiness of political leaders to adopt such policies is a nagging issue. Political leaders are little different than the rest of us; they

.focus primarily on short-term issues to the exclusion of long-term concerns, and they often avoid truly difficult issues that might prevent reelection.[29] There also is some evidence that government policy makers view climate-change risks more like people in industry rather than people who are affiliated with environmental groups and university researchers.[87] This may explain the finding that people don't have much trust in government spending as a way of dealing with climate change.[109] It also may be one way that governments perpetuate a national entitlement to consume fossil fuels for economic growth without regard for the risks to the climate of the entire planet.[24]

To truly address climate change and other environmental risks, governments need to engage constituents fairly, openly, and effectively so citizens will buy into the enormous structural and financial changes required to deter global warming.[110] They also should create goals that reverse the loss of critical environmental resources.[111]

Of course, government policies, incentives, and the like only go so far toward changing behavior.[5] Many people don't respond to incentives, such as offering interest to get people to save money for retirement. Laws also don't stop many human behaviors, as drug use and speeding demonstrate. And policies have mostly failed to do away with crime, educate our children equally across the United States, or prevent our ongoing polluting of Earth. Thus, people and the institutions they have created have to take responsibility, too.

There's another concern about political solutions to some of our behavioral problems. Climate change, like so many other pressing issues, has become politically charged.[112] Many people support or refute climate-change policies depending on the stance of their preferred political parties.[94] If political divisiveness is pervasive, this may hinder beneficial policy making.

Government also may not structure itself to truly tackle global warming. In the United States, for example, the federal government may lack the structure needed to formulate policy from climate-change data before disaster strikes.[19] Apart from the obvious disorder we can expect from failing to have an organized prevention plan, it's quite possible government accountability will worsen further as global warming worsens.

Corporations, businesses, and other institutions have received considerably less scrutiny than government when it comes to climate change. It's quite difficult to assess the functioning of these organizations when the people who respond to researchers' questions are individuals in those organizations who may not accurately represent the entire organization.[96] Moreover, many managers are confused about how best to have their organizations address climate change, given the paucity of guidance and the lack of clarity as yet about how global warming will affect their practices.[113,114] This may be why many corporations have so far done little or nothing to address climate change. One interesting finding, though, is that organizational decision makers in the public sector are more likely than their counterparts in the private sector to have values that transcend their organizations, allowing them to more willingly accept policy measures that care for the environment.[96]

Companies also have varied reasons and means for developing a more ecological agenda, according to the small amount of research on this topic:[115]

- Medium-sized companies seem more nimble than large companies, so it's easier for them to institute wholesale changes that make them more Earth-friendly.
- All companies would benefit from creating new internal structures to learn about and then implement more sustainable behavior.
- Companies also benefit from staff who become change agents and have a leadership style that engages employees in the process of becoming more ecologically aware and active.
- And although external forces, such as laws, provide some motivation for corporate sustainability, companies need their consumers to take greater initiative to demand ecological products.

If we expect corporations to engage in behaviors that prevent climate change, their internal processes will have to merge with our desire to alter our consumption through more sustainable products and practices.

Certainly, there is increasing evidence that corporations and organizations are using "environmental intelligence" to become more sensitive to climate change. This action can help them maintain competitive advantages and prevent the economic shocks to their operations that global warming may engender.[114] The media report almost daily that corporations such as Wal-Mart, Google, and Hewlett-Packard are becoming "greener" through the use of renewable energy, reductions in consumption, or changes to sustainable business practices. Other businesses, such as Alcoa, Dow Chemical, and DuPont, have banded together with organizations as the Global Roundtable on Climate Change to seek solutions to global warming. And an international consortium of corporations that includes Coca-Cola, Shell, and Nestlé has asked governments to set standards for them to attain low-carbon emissions. Although some of these moves may be posturing, corporate behavior is beginning to change to attend to the impending risks of climate change that will affect the bottom line. This could be an indication that these organizations are moving beyond monetary and policy concerns to developing more farsighted socially and ecologically responsible management.

Our institutions of higher education also have been called to task for their role in addressing climate change. They have been accused of downplaying the importance of climate change and using too much energy themselves, hindering their ability to influence global warming policy.[116] Others note that education at all levels—for children, adults, at typical schools, and elsewhere—must become more participatory and creative in the fight against global warming.[21,117,118] It appears that educational efforts work better when they consider not just the imparting of knowledge but also people's emotions, sense of community, and their connection with the natural world around them.[119,120]

The ideal is for individuals to work with their governments, businesses, schools, and organizations so that everyone takes responsibility for tackling climate change.[5] An electorate that is well informed about global warming may be vital to ensuring that political and other institutional processes help to create climate-saving policies that are doable now.[17] That leads us to the next issue: how to communicate to citizens so they want to participate in resolving the climate-change problem.

## Media and Communications

As global warming has become a more pressing matter, news sources, TV and radio talk shows, opinion polls, movies and videos, local political and topical forums, special community advertisements, and many other means of communication have addressed the issue. Ample evidence shows that all of these media can play a real role in shaping human behavior.[121] Thus, effective communication about climate change and its risks might help people to see that their actions affect the world around them, sometimes in profoundly harmful ways, and give them options for changing their behavior.

At its most basic level, the frequency and intensity with which the media address topics such as climate change affect how much people believe such an issue is truly important.[28,39,121] The media tend to focus on topics that become more important through scientific research, with public concern providing a feedback loop that can amplify public perceptions while also amplifying media loudness about risks. So, our levels of concern can be heightened as a result of how media portray these risks as much as by the actual seriousness of the risks themselves.[40]

Good communication also works in other ways. Well-tailored messages to help businesses be more environmentally sound, for example, appear to achieve that result.[122] And effective communication can help over-fearful people remain calm and provide ways to keep safe despite potential risks. Communication really can level the playing field by removing some of the barriers that politics, economics, and other human factors put in the way of action against global warming.[77,121]

With the increasing amounts of data available, media portrayals of climate change have been growing in recent years, even though there is evidence that media and public interest in the issue waxes and wanes.[35,123] Images of and stories about more dangerous storms, melting glaciers, droughts, and heat waves have become more pervasive, as have communications about the science, policy, and business implications surrounding global warming. Importantly, there are differences in how media locally and around the world portray climate change, with some providing more and clearer information and others focusing on topics that may or may not be useful to the public's understanding of the issue.[35,124] Even communicators of risk at government agencies may have different perceptions of their ability to get the message out about such environmental problems as climate change.[125]

Overall, though, it's evident that media and other risk communicators aren't doing a great job of educating us about global warming so that we truly understand why we need to change our behavior.[17,126,127] One impediment is that media seek so-called balance between the pro and con camps on the issue without truly understanding the science underlying the warming planet. This can create ambiguity in messages about climate change, which can harm rational thinking about it.[128] As a side effect, this also has distanced scientists from communicating with the media for fear their messages will be misconstrued or made overly simplistic.

It's also clear that media offer confusing messages about climate change.[129] Part of this may be because the media aren't sure how to present an issue in which the most evident effects seem to be happening far away and that may not hit home for some time. This makes local angles difficult to find.[9,80] Furthermore, messages tend to come in specific forms, ranging from the more common alarmist and pessimistic messages to less common optimistic ones. These polar opposite messages can, as we've discussed earlier, lead to fearful inaction, a sense that nothing needs to change, or an expectation that technology or development will save us.[20,129]

Media also may engender outright distrust.[39,109,130,131] They may fail to filter the complicated language, irrelevant side issues, or personal agendas of scientists, politicians, corporate executives, environmentalists, and others, leading citizens to wonder about the reliability, relevance, and clarity of messages about climate change. In this way, media may be complicit in preventing us from understanding how global warming occurs, how it affects us personally, and what roles we can play in its resolution.[74,126]

Although our perceptions of the risks of climate change are bound to evolve as global warming does more damage, if media are to play a vital role in preventing that harm they must become more trustworthy in their presentation of the facts, make the story relevant to our lives, and give us information about specific things we can do to fight the problem here and now. [44,127,129] Moreover, as global citizens we must become more engaged in sifting through all of the information that is available to determine what is reliable so we can take some responsibility for our own behavior change. Remember personal responsibility and self-efficacy? Some say we need to become "ordinary heroes" to tackle global warming,[129] and we need media that can brand the issue, help us feel positive about making environmentally friendly choices, and connect citizens in this pursuit. We'll talk more about the importance of that connectedness next.

## Social Identity: Norms, Connections, and Movements

People who perceive that they are connected with others, whether it's through cooperation with neighbors or peers to solve problems or by a sense of belonging to supportive networks, are more likely to exhibit interest in ecological activities.[132,133] People who have this social identification benefit not just from the interaction but also from a sense of group cohesion toward solving a problem.

Another form of social influence comes from groups that heighten people's awareness of risks.[28] In addition to media influence, many environmental and other groups communicate among their members about the potential harm caused by climate change, making the problem more immediate and engendering concern. People then pass their concern on to others, creating a social movement about climate change. This movement, or collective action, appears to benefit from the involvement of individuals who have knowledge about the problem and a sense of self-efficacy about the specific actions the group can take to prevent harm.[134] By contrast, people also can be part of a "social malaise," which can prevent ecological behaviors from occurring.[135] Underlying this malaise, often in our cities, are such factors as poverty, deviant behaviors, a lack of social cohesion, and people just doing what they can for themselves to survive.

Given the gaps in the research, it's unclear whether having a sense of social identity would motivate many people to become more active in pursuing collective solutions to climate change, but it's a good bet that it would for some of us. As has already been noted, studies indicate that people who live in communities or cultures with social norms that encourage environmentally friendly practices tend to follow those norms, be they from friends, religious beliefs, education, or other sources. Moreover, people who are focused on justice for their communities—rather than on self-interested economic considerations—when dealing with environmental problems are more likely to demonstrate ecological behavior and support for policies that attend to global warming.[82] If the community's norm is to find ways to prevent climate change from harming people, it's likely that many people will abide by it.

Changing social or cultural norms to be more environmentally sound, however, isn't something that happens easily or quickly. Government and media campaigns don't work well alone, but norms do change in time when such campaigns are combined with targeted efforts to engage and coach key people in communities, demonstrate a sense that collective habits are changing, and provide economic incentives and sanctions.[5]

The level of collective action that people adopt toward climate change also is of interest. Currently, it appears that most of this group action is relatively small, consisting mostly of local activities, protests, and campaigns to influence individuals and power brokers in communities and states. Although a discussion of mass movements, such as those associated with the civil rights and anti-war movements, is beyond this book's purview, it appears that a larger movement to tackle global warming is building in the United States. This movement likely will engage in efforts to motivate individual behavior change as well as seek broad changes in the regulations and practices of government, industry, and other institutions.[105] Climate change is such a terrible risk to our health and the health of our planet that it deserves just such a response.

## Place

Although a sense of connection with others is an important component to ecological behavior, so is a sense of connection with the community—or place—itself. Individual, group, and cultural connectedness to place appears to affect our behavior toward fighting environmental harm. When people live in a place that they know will be harmed by a new power plant, for instance, they are more likely to be upset about it if they're attached to the place.[136] Our attachment to places is essential to our identity and can boost our sense of self and self-efficacy, but it also has the ability to harm those components of our personality.[137,138] Environmental threats to the places we love could either motivate us to act against them or demoralize us into inaction if the threats seem insurmountable.

Research has shown that people who feel connected to the place where they live are more likely to demonstrate interest in behaving in ecological ways.[133,138] Less attachment means less environmentally sustainable behavior.

Regardless of how attached we are to places, the places themselves can either facilitate or impede sustainable behaviors.[135] Bigger cities that lack mass transit, for example, often require more use of individual transport to get around, which fuels $CO_2$ emissions. Other cities may lack green spaces or manage their natural resources poorly, which can prevent people from attaining a sense of connection to nature and the propensity to care about it. Communities that demonstrate little effort to bring people together through housing, opportunities, and activities, or that are downright dangerous or divisive, also may reduce citizens' hope of living well in those places.

Place has other potential effects on our climate-related behavior. Place attachment can lead to "parochialism," which means we favor the places and groups to which we belong more than those that are beyond our experience.[40] One of the concerns about people who are parochial is they may be less interested in helping outsiders. Because climate change is more likely to harm poor people, especially in foreign lands, and because evidence shows that poverty and place combine to increase the risk for people to have behavioral problems,[139] parochial responses to global warming may prevent people from assisting those doubly injured communities. One of the benefits of parochialism, however, is that places can represent social groups with shared values and purposes. In that case, place can motivate people to work together to reduce such risks as climate change.[133]

Finally, you may recall from the discussion about communication that making climate change local—to the places and communities in which we live—can enhance our desire to be involved in fighting this problem.[9] Making global warming relevant to the place where you live can combine with the social identity you have from interacting with people in that place and drive action. Initiatives in your towns and communities that affect local individual, government, and corporate behavior may be quite influential in getting citizens to behave in climate-protective ways.

## Other External Factors

We have covered some of the most influential external factors on our behavior, and there are more. Among them are social class; job opportunities;

cultural styles; religious and spiritual beliefs; and differences among rural, suburban, and urban dwellers. The research that explores the influence of these factors on our environmental behavior has yielded conflicting results.[64]

We don't have the space to address these myriad factors, but let's briefly look at how complicated they can be. If, for example, a factory is polluting a rural community's air and pumping out huge amounts of $CO_2$, that situation provides a clear problem that may require action. But what sort of action to take becomes less clear if most of that community's citizens work in the factory or reap financial benefits from it, if there are few other employment options nearby, and if the community's leaders are related to the factory's managers. Research indicates that when people experience such economic risks, their participation in preventing environmental harm declines.[64]

Unlike the polluting factory scenario, most people don't see strong connections between their behavior and situations in their communities and how their personal and community factors work together to fuel climate change. Many of us don't think much about our political and economic support for the oil and coal industries, our desire to consume more and more, and our disconnection from nature, but these internally and externally motivated behaviors are harming us through global warming and depleting resources. We must ponder all that it will take to change our individual behavior and the behavior of our governments, corporations, organizations, schools, and other institutions to minimize the impact of climate chaos.

## HOPE FOR THE MEETING OF INDIVIDUAL AND COMMUNITY FACTORS

The connections between people and the community factors that affect them are complex. These factors influence our behavior, and we influence theirs. Together we create ways of life that are leading us toward great harm—heat stress, polluted air, insufficient food and clean water, sea-level rise and extreme weather events, infectious disease, and ecosystem disruption. Human and planetary health hang in the balance. None of us will be able to act in a vacuum free from external impediments if climate chaos prevails.

Some say it may be too difficult to motivate individuals, governments, corporations, and other institutions to change their behavior enough to stop climate change.[24,25] But many others say that we have no choice but to begin this effort immediately by changing how we act. To get there, we can't simply change our environmental worldview—with all of the concern, thinking, responsibility, self-efficacy, and risk perception that goes into it—because that doesn't entirely predict our environmental behavior given our automatic thought processes, habits, and external barriers.[85]

Instead, the power to truly deal with global warming lies in pairing individuals with community factors to make the prevention of climate change for our health our primary principle.[19] We will need to summon all that is best about humanity to prevent this life-threatening climate problem of our own making. It will require the sort of effort we've marshaled before to bring an end to world wars, nuclear terror, and other planet-threatening injustices.

## SOLUTIONS

With the disconnection between our brains and our actions and potential community impediments in our way, changing our behavior to prevent climate chaos from becoming a reality is anything but simple. This book, however, is all about helping us to solve global warming before it creates more harm to our health and the well-being of the planet, and researchers believe the following solutions can really help. We've already outlined some of these solutions in this chapter, so we'll be brief in this section as we begin with what you can do as an individual.

### Individual Solutions

- Educate yourself about the real risks that climate change portends.
- Learn about what's now being done in your communities, at the government level, and around the world to prevent climate change.
- Think! Don't allow automatic mental mechanisms, biases, fears, or a short-term perspective to stop you from taking action.
- Evaluate your habits and make specific goals and commitments to live an ecological lifestyle. This will give you a sense of responsibility and efficacy.
- When you act, do more than one thing to fight global warming.
- Increase your contact with nature to enhance your understanding of its relevance to your life and the importance of protecting it.
- Be willing to pay a bit more to be environmentally responsible.
- Reduce your consumption and learn that living with less needn't ruin your lifestyle.
- Be conscious of wasting energy and be more and more energy efficient: Buy energy-efficient appliances, autos, and light bulbs—and use them less.
- Buy locally and sustainably made products.

- Understand that climate change is a health problem that could harm tens of millions of people and the planet that sustains us. Let that understanding motivate you to act.

## Community Solutions

- Foster or join groups in your area that are actively committed to preventing climate change. This will build your sense of community, limit thinking only about yourself, and give you a sense of collective action so you don't feel overwhelmed by—or overanxious about— the barriers that exist. And then you won't just rely on government, institutions, or technology to address global warming.
- Keep it local! Engage in specific tasks with groups in your communities to fight against the potential local effects of global warming, including droughts, floods, and heavy storms. Taking communal action will help you feel that you have some ability to be helpful with the enormous climate-change problem.
- But also engage in international efforts. Find ways to help people and places in foreign lands that are more likely to experience the harm of climate change sooner. Many organizations, such as the American Red Cross, Oxfam, and the World Wildlife Federation, are involved in such efforts, and they may have local offices in your area.
- Petition political and business leaders to implement laws and policies that truly tackle climate change.
- Contact media outlets, demanding that they provide better information about the effects of climate change and what people can do to prevent them.
- Work with school leaders and teachers to develop teaching tools that will help children and adults to better understand the implications of global warming and what we must do to deter it.

We've discussed how the people who oversee our economic development, government officials, corporate leaders, scientists, and other institutional leaders must take more action on global warming themselves for the benefit of us all. This next section speaks to what they can do.

- If you're an economist or have a hand in how our economy functions, take into account all the costs of climate change, take a far-sighted approach to its risks, realize that economic growth may not prevent it, and seek ways to ensure that economic development and sustainability work together rather than at odds with each other.

- If you play a role in governing and policy making at the local, state, or national level, it's time to use climate-change data to create and enact policies focused on reducing its risks for the people you serve. Make more of an effort to include citizens and organizations in the process of developing cost-effective, trustworthy, and just methods to deter global warming. Oh, and drop the political posturing that prevents action on this important matter!
- If you work in local government and see that national officials are failing to lead, step up and make local policy that deters climate change for the people you represent. It's an important start.
- If you work in a corporation, become a leader—a change agent—for creating environmentally sustainable business practices. Find ways to reduce corporate consumption, produce products that don't overtax our resources or harm our environment, and make the well-being of your customers your primary principle.
- Move your corporation or business in the direction of greater openness to work with consumers and their communities to create a culture of sustainability and reduced resource consumption.
- Corporations and businesses have a lot more clout to influence governments, economies, and communities when they join together to persuade citizens that environmental care is essential to stave off climate chaos.
- If you work in any form of media, there is no time to waste becoming more informed and more trustworthy about the realities of global warming so you can communicate about it more effectively.
- And the way you communicate the risks requires more scrutiny. Are you tailoring the information in ways that inform and motivate citizens and power brokers to engage in activities that actually do something about preventing climate change's potential harm?
- Advertisers, a media subset, also should become more involved in and better at branding global warming and selling solutions to its risks.
- If you're a scientist who plays a role in climate-change issues, it's important for you to communicate about global warming and its health risks in ways that people truly understand.
- Scientists also need to move beyond focusing only on the science of the problem. They also need to use their knowledge to propose specific doable behaviors that individuals, governments, and institutions can adopt to prevent the risks we're facing from climate change. Scientific research must inform public policy.
- If you represent people in local communities, take the time to outline for your citizens the expected norms for more sustainable lifestyles. This may require providing more options when it comes to energy efficiency, increasing access

to healthy local food resources, offering recycling facilities, and developing related activities that can help people reduce their consumption and be better stewards of the places in which they live.

- Place is vitally important in ecological behavior, and community leaders and citizens should expend the energy to improve the quality of their places so that we feel compelled to care for them in sustainable ways. Doing this can combat social malaise and make for safer communities, too.
- Educators also must step up and become more involved in this endeavor, using all modern means available and their connections with their communities to teach about climate change and how to prevail against it.
- Finally, we all benefit from feedback—from knowing how well individual energy-saving behavior is going to how well media are influencing that behavior.[7,140] When we know that our perspectives are understood, believe that our right to choose is respected, and understand why our choices may have to be motivated or restricted to deter climate chaos, it will go a long way to encouraging us to behave more ecologically.[141]

Preventing climate chaos is possible if all of these factors work together to create opportunities and policies locally and around the world to save our planet from what we humans have wrought.[142] There is evidence that the rise of international efforts to prevent environmental degradation has demonstrated some success. Those efforts work best when they receive support and guidance, use good communication to accomplish their goals, and remain persistent over time.[143] If we change our behavior, we can clearly prevent climate chaos.

# Chapter 11

## Epilogue

Maria knows this isn't any ordinary day. Her family has been through a lot, just like millions of other families and thousands of communities around the United States and the world that have been striving for years to turn the tide against climate change. But today the United Nations is hosting an International Climate Celebration in communities all over the Earth to pay tribute to the worldwide efforts that have changed the course of the climate for the better—for the planet and all its living creatures. Finally, greenhouse gas emissions have fallen to historic lows, and the planetary warming and its harm are declining.

It all began, of course, when enough people awoke to the reality of the scientists' data that showed climate change really was heating the planet and causing more droughts and heat waves; devastating storms and floods, hurricanes and tornadoes; water and food shortages; soaring infectious disease rates; plant and animal extinctions; and, ultimately, illness, displacement, and misery for millions of Earth's citizens. Then, fast-declining oil reserves and the scramble to use coal energy in its place made the climate even less stable. A small movement started with a handful of individuals, some local community groups, a few larger organizations and businesses, and a minority of politicians and powerbrokers around the world who were concerned about what climate change and insufficient clean energy options could mean for Earth's very existence.

As the damage to people and the planet mounted, more and more people began to cry out that action had to happen—and now. We set aside our limited automatic thinking, our entrenched ways of living, and our desire to mostly meet our own needs rather than the needs of our fellow citizens and our only planet. We began to call for concerted action. We joined groups and pushed for legislation—locally, nationally, and internationally—to implement solutions, offer incentives, and find common ground to reduce our greenhouse gas emissions and live more sustainable lifestyles.

A host of solutions were put into place: renewable energy, energy efficiency, use of fewer resources, recycling everything, and smaller homes and tighter communities with less sprawl. We began to live, work, and produce products closer to home to reduce unnecessary travel and shipping. We adopted locally based organic agriculture—even in people's own backyards and nearby parks—and less meat consumption. We began to care for the vulnerable close to home and far away.

Cooperative agreements amid nations and corporations sprang up, with incentives, guidelines, and clear lines of responsibility for ecological action. Businesses actually asked for government standards and oversight by which to operate so their long-range business plans could include projected costs, fees, and taxes to avoid the full range of climate surprises. They also harnessed technology to strive toward efficiency when they realized how much money could be saved while improving the climate in the process.

Economists and money brokers also reconfigured their models to downplay the value of ceaseless competition for more profits—at the cost of the climate and our social fabric—and instead adopted a model that recognized that the planet has finite resources, that growth cannot solve all problems, and that sustainability and the fair distribution of goods and services are truly humane economic goals. Media, meanwhile, worked harder to communicate the realities of the climate horrors and focused on tailored messages that directed people and their institutions to specific behavior changes so that everyone could participate to prevent climate chaos. Education led in finding new ways to teach people of all ages and persuasions about the climate, the planet, and our role as Earth's stewards for our own health and destinies. And people and the institutions they created used all of these methods and more to behave differently toward Earth and its limited but invaluable resources. We began to actually care for it, nurture it, and live in balance with it.

Maria remembers how her family members chose to rely on more local products and to live more simply and more in tune with the world around them. That meant buying organic food from nearby farms rather than food from across the globe. That meant driving less and in fuel-efficient cars or, better yet, Moravia telecommuting to work and everyone taking mass transit to engage in family activities away from home. It meant conserving energy at home by going without so many electronic extras, cutting back on energy use, and putting in new high-efficiency appliances. It meant working with local activists to take care of the elderly, children, and the poor to make it through some of the hot, air-polluted days and the times when water and food were scarce, which still occurr but less often now. It meant learning to work hard every day to reduce consumption, despite the stresses on the family, and embracing a changing economic system that had dropped its growth-at-all-costs, profit-making motives in favor of husbanding Earth and its resources so everyone could survive the life-threatening climate and energy problems people had created.

Maria participated in all of this. She participated in efforts that helped enlighten people about the damage their consumerism was doing to the planet. She participated in showing individuals, institutions, businesses, and governments the reality of the enormous and devastating costs inherent in using fossil fuels to move food and other products across the planet; to power our homes, cars, and businesses; and to maintain good lifestyles for the few when billions lived in poverty. And she participated in helping the planet move in new directions, one of the most promising being the United Nations' unanimous declaration that the health of Earth's citizens, creatures, and resources was the primary principle on which all decisions—political, economic, and social—must be based as we became caretakers of a sustainable, caring, and just new world.

Certainly, there still are struggles, Maria now thinks. Climate change has not yet fully abated. Many miles of former coastline and their communities remain submerged. Air quality still often suffers. Water quality and quantity are persistent problems in many places, and sometimes food shortages occur with the variable weather (although now food and water distribution efforts that use as little energy as possible are rapid, efficient affairs that keep almost everyone well sustained around the globe). Some of her elderly patients still have more health woes than before global warming began, but they aren't dying quite as readily from the heat and the stress. It simply isn't as bad as some had predicted it would get—before people and their institutions began to make wholesale changes in the way they behaved toward climate change in the world around them.

Maria also sees that her children and siblings are faring so much better as global warming has begun to abate. Zach's asthma isn't nearly as bad as it had been. Max and Magda and their families are less stressed and have built new, happier, sustainable lives not far from Maria's home. They get together often, reconnecting in ways that don't rely on their former lifestyles based on consumerism. Instead they cherish the shared purpose of making their love and appreciation for one another stronger and their community better for everyone.

Maria smiles steadily for the first time in years. She's getting on a community shuttle bus with Moravia and her kids to go to the United Nations Celebration at the city center. People are bringing homemade goodies created from locally grown produce. They're coming with blankets and lawn chairs to celebrate together their vital roles in the local and global efforts that have reduced climate-changing emissions. But they'll also be partying with millions of their fellow citizens from communities around the world via a low-energy satellite link broadcast that will be shown on flat-panel screens so that millions of people can be with each other at this truly worldwide, multinational gathering of joyous humanity. It will be a day without conflict, a day to share, a day to honor the human capacity to save itself from the harm that it had created before it knew the truth and took action.

Unlike the other tale of Maria and her family that has led you through Climate Chaos, we leave you with this other story of Maria. This is our hopeful vision of our planet's future. We have a choice. Let's choose this ending.

# References

## CHAPTER 2

1. IPCC, 2007: *Summary for Policymakers*. In: Solomon S, Qin D, Manning M, Chen Z, Marquis M, Averyt KB, et al., editors. *Climate Change 2007: The Physical Science Basis. Contribution of Working Group I to the Fourth Assessment Report of the Intergovernmental Panel on Climate Change*. Cambridge, United Kingdom, and New York: Cambridge University Press; 2007.

2. World Meteorological Organization. Press Release No. 805, 2007.

3. Gutro R. 2005. Warmest Year in Over a Century. 2006; Available at: http://www.nasa.gov/vision/earth/environment/2005_warmest.html Accessed 1/6/2008.

4. Goswami BN, Venugopal V, Sengupta D, Madhusoodanan MS, Xavier PK. Increasing Trend of Extreme Rain Events over India in a Warming Environment. *Science* 2006; 314:1442–1445.

5. U.S. Global Change Research Information Office. What Is the Greenhouse Effect? 1996; Available at: http://www.gcrio.org/ocp96/p30box.html Accessed 12/29/2007.

6. Flannery T. *The Weather Makers: How Man Is Changing the Climate and What It Means for Life on Earth*. New York: Atlantic Monthly Press; 2005.

7. U.S. Environmental Protection Agency. Climate Change 2007; Available at: http://www.epa.gov/climatechange/index.html Accessed 12/29/2007.

8. Williams DR. Moon Fact Sheet 2006; Available at: http://nssdc.gsfc.nasa.gov/planetary/factsheet/moonfact.html Accessed 12/8/2007.

9. Stute M, Forster M, Frischkorn H, Serejo A, Clark JF, Schlosser P, et al. Cooling of Tropical Brazil (5°C) During the Last Glacial Maximum. *Science* 1995; 269:379–383.

10. Hansen J, Sato M, Kharecha P, Russell G, Lea DW, Siddall M. Climate Change and Trace Gases. *Philosophical Transactions of the Royal Society A*. 2007; 365(1925):1954.

11. Solomon S, Qin D, Manning M, Alley RB, Berntsen T, Bindoff NL, et al. *Technical Summary.* In: Solomon S, Qin D, Manning M, Chen Z, Marquis M, Averyt KB, et al., editors. *Climate Change 2007: The Physical Science Basis. Contribution of Working Group I to the Fourth Assessment Report of the Intergovernmental Panel on Climate Change.* Cambridge, United Kingdom, and New York: Cambridge University Press; 2007.

12. Stern N. The Stern Review Report on the Economics of Climate Change. 2006. Available at: http://www.hm-treasury.gov.uk/independent_reviews/stern_review_economics_climate_change/stern_review_report.cfm Accessed 1/31/2008.

13. Office of Transportation and Air Quality, U.S. Environmental Protection Agency. Mobile Source Emissions—Past, Present, and Future. 2007; Available at: http://www.epa.gov/otaq/invntory/overview/pollutants/nox.htm#onroad Accessed 12/30/2007.

14. U. S. National Academy of Sciences, National Research Council Committee on Abrupt Climate Change. *Abrupt Climate Change: Inevitable Surprises.* 2002.

15. Cunningham SA, Kanzow T, Rayner D, Baringer MO, Johns WE, Marotzke J, et al. Temporal Variability of the Atlantic Meridional Overturning Circulation at 26.5°N. *Science* 2007; 317(5840): 935–938.

16. Baumert KA, Herzog T, Markoff M. Climate Analysis Indicators Tool (CAIT) Version 5.0. 2007; Available at: http://cait.wri.org/ Accessed 1/5/2008.

## CHAPTER 3

1. Stott PA, Stone DA, Allen MR. Human Contribution to the European Heatwave of 2003. *Nature* 2004; 432:610–614.

2. National Climatic Data Center. Climate of 2007—in Historical Perspective: Preliminary Annual Report. 2007; Available at: http://www.ncdc.noaa.gov/oa/climate/research/2007/ann/ann07.html NOAA Satellite and Information Service. Accessed 1/6/2008.

3. Centers for Disease Control. Heat-Related Illnesses, Deaths, and Risk Factors—Cincinnati and Dayton, Ohio, 1999, and United States, 1979–1997. *Morbidity and Mortality Weekly Report* 2000; 49(21):470–473.

4. Solomon S, Qin D, Manning M, Alley RB, Berntsen T, Bindoff NL, et al. *Technical Summary.* In: Solomon S, Qin D, Manning M, Chen Z, Marquis M, Averyt KB, et al, editors. *Climate Change 2007: The Physical Science Basis. Contribution of Working Group I to the Fourth Assessment Report of the Intergovernmental Panel on Climate Change.* Cambridge. United Kingdom, and New York: Cambridge University Press; 2007.

5. Goddard Institute for Space Studies. NASA Study Suggests Extreme Summer Warming in the Future. 2007; Available at: http://www.giss.nasa.gov/research/news/20070509/ National Aeronautics and Space Agency. Accessed 1/6/2008.

6. Semenza JC, Rubin CH, Falter KH, Selanikio JD, Flanders WD, Howe HL, et al. Heat-Related Deaths during the July 1995 Heat Wave in Chicago. *The New England Journal of Medicine* 1996; 335(2):84–90.

7. Kosatsky T. The 2003 European Heat Waves. *Eurosurveillance* 2005; 10(7):148–149.

8. Della-Marta PM, Haylock MR, Luterbacher J, Wanner H. Doubled Length of Western European Summer Heat Waves Since 1880. *Journal of Geophysical Research* 2007; 112:doi:10.1029/2007JD008510.

9. Rogers JC, Wang S, Coleman, Jill SM. Evaluation of a Long-Term (1882–2005) Equivalent Temperature Time Series. *Journal of Climate* 2007; 20(17):4476–4485.

10. Rooney C, McMichael AJ, Kovats RS, Coleman MP. Excess Mortality in England and Wales, and in Greater London, During the 1995 Heatwave. *Journal of Epidemiology and Community Health* 1998; 52:482–486.

11. Ogawa T. *Heat Disorders*. In: Stellman JM, editor. *Encyclopaedia of Occupational Health and Safety*. Fourth ed. Hamilton, Ontario: International Labor Office; 1998, pp. 1–6.

12. Bouchama A. The 2003 European Heat Wave. *Intensive Care Medicine* 2004; 30:1–3.

13. Belmin J, Auffray J, Berbezier C, Boirin P, Mercier S, de Reviers B, et al. Level of Dependency: A Simple Marker Associated with Mortality during the 2003 Heatwave among French Dependent Elderly People Living in the Community or in Institutions. *Age and Ageing* 2007; 36(3):298–303.

14. Semenza JC, Krishnasamy PV. Design of a Health-Promoting Neighborhood Intervention. *Health Promotion Practice* 2007; 8(3):243–256.

15. Nunneley S. *Prevention of Heat Stress*. In: Stellman JM, editor. *Encyclopaedia of Occupational Health and Safety*. Fourth ed. Hamilton, Ontario: International Labor Office; 1998, pp. 1–7.

16. Hales S, Edwards SJ, Kovats RS. *Impacts on Health of Climate Extremes*. In: McMichael AJ, Campbell-Lendrum DH, Corvalan CF, Ebi KL, Githeko AK, Scheraga JD, et al, editors. *Climate Change and Human Health: Risks and Responses*. Geneva: World Health Organization; 2003, pp. 79–102.

17. Nag PK, Nag A, Ashtekar SP. Thermal Limits of Men in Moderate to Heavy Work in Tropical Farming. *Industrial Health* 2007; 45:107–117.

18. National Center for Children in Poverty. Basic Facts About Low-Income Children: Birth to Age 6. 2007. Columbia University Mailman School of Public Health, New York. Available at: http://www.nccp.org/publications/pdf/download_215.pdf Accessed 5/17/2008.

19. U.S. Census Bureau. People: Poverty. 2004; Available at: http://factfinder.census.gov/jsp/saff/SAFFInfo.jsp?_pageId=tp8_poverty Accessed 1/5/2008.

20. Huntingford C, Hemming D, Gash JHC, Gedney N, Nuttall PA. Impact of Climate Change on Health: What is Required of Climate Modellers? *Transactions of the Royal Society of Tropical Medicine and Hygiene* 2007; 101:97–103.

21. Conti S, Meli P, Minelli G, Solimini R, Toccaceli V, Vichi M, et al. Epidemiologic Study of Mortality during the Summer 2003 Heat Wave in Italy. *Environmental Research* 2005; 98:390–399.

22. Hajat S, Kovats RS, Lachowycz K. Heat-Related and Cold-Related Deaths in England and Wales: Who Is at Risk? *Occupational and Environmental Medicine* 2007; 64(2):93–100.

23. Basu R, Samet JM. Relation between Elevated Ambient Temperature and Mortality: A Review of the Epidemiologic Evidence. *Epidemiologic Reviews* 2002; 24(2):190–202.

24. Whitman S, Good G, Donoghue ER, Benbow N, Shou W, Mou S. Mortality in Chicago Attributed to the July 1995 Heat Wave. *American Journal of Public Health* 1997; 87(9):1515–1518.

25. Lowen AC, Mubareka S, Steel J, Palese P. Influenza Virus Transmission Is Dependent on Relative Humidity and Temperature. *PLoS Pathogens* 2007; 3(10):e151.

26. Bulbena A, Sperry L, Cunillera J. Psychiatric Effects of Heat Waves. *Psychiatric Services* 2006; 57(10):1519–1519.

27. Nitschke M, Tucker GR, Bi P. Morbidity and Mortality during Heatwaves in Metropolitan Adelaide. *Medical Journal of Australia* 2007; 187(11/12):662–665.

28. Bell PA. Reanalysis and Perspective in the Heat-Aggression Debate. *Journal of Personality and Social Psychololgy* 2005; 89:71–73.

29. Rotton J, Cohn EG. Global Warming and U.S. Crime Rates: An Application of Routine Activity Theory. *Environment and Behavior* 2003; 35:802–825.

30. Rotton J, Frey J. Air Pollution, Weather, and Violent Crimes: Concomitant Time-Series Analysis of Archival Data. *Journal of Personality and Social Psychology* 1985; 49(5):1207–1220.

31. Simister J, Cooper C. Thermal Stress in the U.S.A.: Effects on Violence and on Employee Behaviour. *Stress and Health: Journal of the International Society for the Investigation of Stress* 2005; 21:3–15.

32. Anderson CA. Heat and Violence. *Current Directions in Psychological Science* 2001; 10:33–38.

33. Bushman BJ, Wang MC, Anderson CA. Is the Curve Relating Temperature to Aggression Linear or Curvilinear? Assaults and Temperature in Minneapolis Reexamined. *Journal of Personality and Social Psychology* 2005; 89:62–66.

34. Kuo FE, Sullivan WC. Environment and Crime in the Inner City: Does Vegetation Reduce Crime? *Environment and Behavior* 2001; 33(3):343–367.

35. ———. Aggression and Violence in the Inner City: Effects of Environment via Mental Fatigue. *Environment and Behavior* 2001; 33(4):543–571.

36. Kellermann AL, Todd KH. Killing Heat. *New England Journal of Medicine* 1996; 335(2):126–127.

37. Ebi KL, Teisberg TJ, Kalkstein LS, Robinson L, Weiher RF. Heat Watch/Warning Systems Save Lives: Estimated Costs and Benefits for Philadelphia 1995–98. *American Meteorological Society* 2004:1067–1073.

38. Bernard SM, McGeehin MA. Municipal Heat Wave Response Plans. *American Journal of Public Health* 2004; 94(9):1520–1522.

39. City of Chicago. Green Roofs Open to the Public. 2006; Available at: http://64.233.169.104/search?q=cache:UllVmAn5f9kJ:www.cityofchicago.org/environment+chicago+green+roofs&hl=en&ct=clnk&cd=2&gl=us Accessed 1/5/2008.

# CHAPTER 4

1. West JJ, Fiore AM, Horowitz LW, Mauzerall DL. Global Health Benefits of Mitigating Ozone Pollution with Methane Emission Controls. *Proceedings of the National Academy of Sciences* 2006; 103(11):3988–3993.

2. Shindell D. Understanding Carbon Monoxide as Pollutant and as Agent of Climate Change. 2007; Available at: http://www.giss.nasa.gov/research/briefs/shindell_09/ NASA Goddard Institute for Space Studies. Accessed 1/10/2008.

3. Knowlton K, Rosenthal JE, Hogrefe C, Lynn B, Gaffin S, Gore F, et al. Assessing Ozone-Related Health Impacts under a Changing Climate. *Environmental Health Perspectives* 2004; 112(15):1557–1563.

4. Bell ML, Goldberg R, Hogrefe C, Kinney PL, Knowlton K, Lynn B, et al. Climate Change, Ambient Ozone, and Health in 50 US Cities. *Climatic Change* 2007; 82(1–2).

5. McConnell R, Berhane K, Gilliland F, London SJ, Islam T, Gauderman WJ, et al. Asthma in Exercising Children Exposed to Ozone: A Cohort Study. *The Lancet* 2002; 359(9304):386–391.

6. Hathout EH, Beeson WL, Ischander M, Rao R, Mace JW. Air Pollution and Type 1 Diabetes in Children. *Pediatric Diabetes* 2006; 7:81–87.

7. Schwartz J. Air Pollution and Children's Health. *Pediatrics* 2004; 113(4 Suppl):1037–1043.

8. Lacour SA, de Monte M, Diot P, Brocca J, Veron N, Colin P, et al. Relationship between Ozone and Temperature during the 2003 Heat Wave in France: Consequences for Health Data Analysis. *BMC Public Health* 2006; 6:261.

9. Filleul L, Cassadou S, Medina S, Fabres P, Lefranc A, Eilstein D, et al. The Relation between Temperature, Ozone, and Mortality in Nine French Cities during the Heat Wave of 2003. *Environmental Health Perspectives* 2006; 114(9):1344–1347.

10. Penn State Milton S. Hershey Medical Center College of Medicine. Gender May Play Role in Recovery from Pneumonia after Ozone Exposure. *Science Daily* 2007; June 26.

11. Maitre A, Bonneterre V, Huillard L, Sabatier P, de Gaudemaris R. Impact of Urban Atmospheric Pollution on Coronary Disease. *European Heart Journal* 2006; 27(19):2275–2284.

12. Gauderman WJ, Vora H, McConnell R, Berhane K, Gilliland F, Thomas D, et al. Effect of Exposure to Traffic on Lung Development from 10 to 18 Years of Age: A Cohort Study. *The Lancet* 2007; 369(9561):571–577.

13. Flanner MG, Zender CS, Randerson JT, Rasch PJ. Present-day Climate Forcing and Response from Black Carbon in Snow. *Journal of Geophysical Research* 2007; 112.

14. Eftim SE, McDermott A, Breysse PN, Samet JM, Geyh A. Canada Forest Fires, Transboundary Air Pollution and Hospitalizations among the Elderly in the Northeastern USA in July 2002. Unpublished data.

15. Flannery T. *The Weather Makers: How Man Is Changing the Climate and What It Means for Life on Earth.* New York: Atlantic Monthly Press; 2005.

16. Pratt GC, Palmer K, Wu CY, Oliaei F, Hollerback C, Fenske MJ. An Assessment of Air Toxics in Minnesota. *Environmental Health Perspectives* 2000; 108(9):815–825.

17. Johnson ES, Langard S, Lin Y. A Critique of Benzene Exposure in the General Population. *Science of the Total Environment* 2007; 374:183–198.

18. Ziska LH, Gebhard DE, Frenz DA, Faulkner S, Singer BD, Straka JG. Cities as Harbingers of Climate Change: Common Ragweed, Urbanization, and Public Health. *Journal of Allergy and Clinical Immunology* 2003; 111(2):290–295.

19. Beggs PJ, Bambrick HJ. Is the Global Rise of Asthma an Early Impact of Anthropogenic Climate Change? *Environmental Health Perspectives* 2005; 113(8):915–919.

20. Yamazaki S, Nitta H, Fukuhara S. Associations Between Exposure to Ambient Photochemical Oxidants and the Vitality or Mental Health Domain of the Health Related Quality of Life. *Journal of Epidemiology & Community Health* 2006; 60:173–179.

21. Chattopadhyay PK, Som B, Mukhopadhyay P. Air Pollution and Health Hazards in Human Subjects: Physiological and Self-Report Indices. *Journal of Environmental Psychology* 1995; 15:327–331.

22. Jacobs SV, Evans GW, Catalano R, Dooley D. Air Pollution and Depressive Symptomatology: Exploratory Analyses of Intervening Psychosocial Factors. *Population & Environment: Behavioral & Social Issues* 1984; 7:260–272.

23. Day RJ. Traffic-Related Air Pollution and Perceived Health Risk: Lay Assessment of an Everyday Hazard. *Health Risk and Society* 2006; 8(3):305–322.

24. Katon W, Lozano P, Russo J, McCauley E, Richardson L, Bush T. The Prevalence of DSM-IV Anxiety and Depressive Disorders in Youth with Asthma Compared with Controls. *Journal of Adolescent Health* 2007; 41(5):455–463.

25. Berz JB. 2007. A Longitudinal Analysis of Asthma, SES, and Socioemotional Functioning during Early Childhood. PhD diss., University of Massachusetts, Boston.

26. Ng T, Chiam P, Kua E. Mental Disorders and Asthma in the Elderly: A Population-Based Study. *International Journal of Geriatric Psychiatry* 2007; 22(7):668–674.

27. Pedersen CB, Raaschou-Nielsen O, Hertel O, Mortensen PB. Air Pollution from Traffic and Schizophrenia Risk. *Schizophrenia Research* 2004; 66(1):83–85.

28. Margai F, Henry N. A Community-Based Assessment of Learning Disabilities Using Environmental and Contextual Risk Factors. *Social Science & Medicine* 2003; 56(5):1073–1085.

29. Rotton J, Frey J. Air Pollution, Weather, and Violent Crimes: Concomitant Time-Series Analysis of Archival Data. *Journal of Personality and Social Psychology* 1985; 49(5):1207–1220.

30. Myers GJ, Davidson PW, Weitzman M, Lanphear BP. Contribution of Heavy Metals to Developmental Disabilities in Children. *Mental Retardation & Developmental Disabilities Research Reviews* 1997; 3(3):239–245.

## CHAPTER 5

1. Solomon S, Qin D, Manning M, Alley RB, Berntsen T, Bindoff NL, et al. *Technical Summary*. In: Solomon S, Qin D, Manning M, Chen Z, Marquis M, Averyt KB, et al., editors. *Climate Change 2007: The Physical Science Basis. Contribution of Working Group 1 to the Fourth Assessment Report of the Intergovernmental Panel on Climate Chage*. Cambridge. United Kingdom, and New York: Cambridge University Press; 2007.

2. Postel SL. Entering an Era of Water Scarcity: The Challenges Ahead. *Ecological Applications* 2000; 10(4):941–948.

3. United States Geological Survey. Estimated Use of Water in the United States in 2000. 2007; Available at: http://pubs.usgs.gov/circ/2004/circ1268/htdocs/text-total.html Accessed 01/28/2008.

4. United Nations Environment Programme. GEO-2000: Global Environment Outlook. 1999; Available at: http://www.unep.org/geo2000/ Accessed 01/31/2008.

5. Kansas Geological Survey. High Plains Ogallala Aquifer Information. 2007; Available at: http://www.epa.gov/region07/education_resources/teachers/activities/wateractivity2.htm Accessed 01/28/2008.

6. Gelt J. Land Subsidence, Earth Fissures Change Arizona's Landscape. *Arroyo* 1992; 6(2). Available at: http://ag.arizona.edu/azwater/arroyo/062land.html Accessed 5/17/2008.

7. Watkins K (lead author). Human Development Report 2006, Beyond Scarcity: Power, Poverty and the Global Water Crisis. 2006. United Nations Development Programme. Available at: http://hdr.undp.org/en/reports/global/hdr2006/ Accessed 01/31/2008.

8. American Water Works Association. Water Use Statistics. 2007; Available at: http://www.drinktap.org/consumerdnn/Default.aspx?tabid=85 Accessed 1/28/2008.

9. Moon BK. A Climate Culprit in Darfur. *Washington Post*; June 16, 2007:A15.

10. Westerling AL, Hidalgo HG, Cayan DR, Swetnam TW. Warming and Earlier Spring Increase Western U.S. Forest Wildfire Activity. *Science* 2006; 313:940–943.

11. Magrin G, García CG, Choque DC, Giménez JC, Moreno AR, Nagy GJ, et al. *2007: Latin America*. In: Parry ML, Canziani OF, Palutikof JP, van der Linden, P.J., Hanson CE, editors. *Climate Change 2007: Impacts, Adaptation and*

*Vulnerability. Contribution of Working Group II to the Fourth Assessment Report of the Intergovernmental Panel on Climate Change.* Cambridge, UK: Cambridge University Press; 2007, pp. 581–615.

12. Mote PW. Climate-Driven Variability and Trends in Mountain Snowpack in Western North America. *Journal of Climate* 2006; 19:6209–6220.

13. Cruz RV, Harasawa H, Lal M, Wu S, Anokhin Y, Púnsalmaa B, et al. *2007: Asia.* In: Parry, ML; Canziani, OF; Palutikof, JP; van der Linden, PJ; Hanson, CE, editors. *Climate Change 2007: Impacts, Adaptation and Vulnerability. Contribution of Working Group II to the Fourth Assessment Report of the Intergovernmental Panel on Climate Change.* Cambridge, UK: Cambridge University Press; 2007.

14. Burke EJ, Brown SJ, Christidis N. Modeling the Recent Evolution of Global Drought and Projections for the Twenty-First Century with the Hadley Centre Climate Model. *Journal of Hydrometeorology* 2006; 7(5):1113–1125.

15. California Coastal Commission. Seawater Desalination and the California Coastal Act. A report to the California Coastal Commission, State of California, Sacramento, CA, March 2004.

16. Christiansen BA. Bottled Water: Better Than the Tap? *FDA Consumer Magazine*, July–August 2002.

17. Larsen J. Bottled Water Boycotts: Back-to-the-Tap Movement Gains Momentum. 2007; Available at: http://www.earth-policy.org/Updates/2007/Update68.htm Earth Policy Institute. Accessed 01/29/2008.

18. Rijsberman F, Mohammed A. Water, Food and Environment: Conflict or Dialogue? *Water, Science & Technology* 2003; 47(6):53–62.

19. Urban Water Conflicts: An Analysis of the Origins and Nature of Water-Related Unrest and Conflicts in the Urban Context. Report No. SC-2006/WS/19:1–188 to the United Nations Educational, Scientific, and Cultural Organization: International Hydrological Programme 2006.

20. Vlachos E. Towards a Typology of Water-Related Conflicts in the Urban Environment. *Water, Science & Technology* 2003; 47(6):205–210.

21. Corral-Verdugo V, Bechtel RB, Fraijo-Sing B. Environmental Beliefs and Water Conservation: An Empirical Study. *Journal of Environmental Psychology* 2003; 23(3):247–257.

22. Corral-Verdugo V, Frías-Armenta M. Personal Normative Beliefs, Antisocial Behavior, and Residential Water Conservation. *Environment and Behavior* 2006; 38(3):406–421.

23. Routhe AS, Jones RE, Feldman DL. Using Theory to Understand Public Support for Collective Actions that Impact the Environment: Alleviating Water Supply Problems in a Nonarid Biome. *Social Science Quarterly* 2005; 86(4):874–897.

24. Van Vugt M, Samuelson CD. The Impact of Personal Metering in the Management of a Natural Resource Crisis: A Social Dilemma Analysis. *Personality and Social Psychology Bulletin* 1999; 25(6):731–745.

25. Forsyth DR, Garcia M, Zyzniewski LE, Story PA, Kerr NA. Watershed Pollution and Preservation: The Awareness-Appraisal Model of Environmentally

Positive Intentions and Behaviors. *Analyses of Social Issues and Public Policy (ASAP)* 2004; 4(1):115–128.

26. de Oliver M. Attitudes and Inaction: A Case Study of the Manifest Demographics of Urban Water Conservation. *Environment and Behavior* 1999; 31(3):372–394.

27. Sartore G, Kelly B, Stain HJ. Drought and Its Effect on Mental Health. *Australian Family Physician* 2007; 36(12):990–993.

28. Coêlho AEL, Adair JG, Mocellin JSP. Psychological Responses to Drought in Northeastern Brazil. *Revista Interamericana de Psicología* 2004; 38(1):95–103.

29. Dean J, Stain HJ. The Impact of Drought on the Emotional Well-Being of Children and Adolescents in Rural and Remote New South Wales. *The Journal of Rural Health* 2007; 23(4):356–364.

30. Shirreffs SM, Merson SJ, Fraser SM, Archer DT. The Effects of Fluid Restriction on Hydration Status and Subjective Feelings in Man. *British Journal of Nutrition* 2004; 91:951–958.

31. Szinnai G, Schachinger H, Arnaud MJ, Linder L, Keller U. Effect of Water Deprivation on Cognitive-Motor Performance in Healthy Men and Women. *American Journal of Physiology-Regulatory, Integrative and Comparative Physiology* 2005; 289:275–280.

32. DeLorme DE, Hagen SC, Stout IJ. Consumers' Perspectives on Water Issues: Directions for Educational Campaigns. *Journal of Environmental Education* 2003; 34(2):28–35.

# CHAPTER 6

1. Assanangkornchai S, Tangboonngam S, Sam-angsri N, Edwards JG. A Thai Community's Anniversary Reaction to a Major Catastrophe. *Stress and Health: Journal of the International Society for the Investigation of Stress* 2007; 23(1):43–50.

2. Kshirsagar NA, Shinde RR, Mehta S. Floods in Mumbai: Impact of Public Health Service by Hospital Staff and Medical Students. *Journal of Postgraduate Medicine* 2006; 52(4):312–314.

3. Ahern M, Kovats RS, Wilkinson P, Few R, Matthies F. Global Health Impacts of Floods: Epidemiologic Evidence. *Epidemiologic Reviews* 2005; 27:36–46.

4. Abramson D, Garfield R. On the Edge: Children and Families Displaced by Hurricanes Katrina and Rita Face a Looming Medical and Mental Health Crisis. A Report of the Louisiana Child & Family Health Study. 2006 (Revised: December 23, 2006). New York: Columbia University, Mailman School of Public Health.

5. Mailman Study Finds Families Displaced by Katrina Still Face Health, Economic Woes. *Association of Schools of Public Health Friday Letter*; 1450:02/07/2007.

6. Madsen T, Figdor E. When It Rains, It Pours: Global Warming and the Rising Frequency of Extreme Precipitation in the United States. Report to Environment America Research and Policy Center 2007; 1–48.

7. Centers for Disease Control and Prevention (CDC). Norovirus Outbreak among Evacuees from Hurricane Katrina—Houston, Texas, September 2005. *MMWR Morbidity and Mortality Weekly Report* 2005; 54(40):1016–1018.

8. Curriero FC, Patz JA, Rose JB, Lele S. The Association between Extreme Precipitation and Waterborne Disease Outbreaks in the United States, 1948–1994. *American Journal of Public Health* 2001; 91(8):1194–1199.

9. Rao CY, Riggs MA, Chew GL, Muilenberg ML, Thorne PS, Van Sickle D, et al. Characterization of Airborne Molds, Endotoxins, and Glucans in Homes in New Orleans after Hurricanes Katrina and Rita. *Applied and Environmental Microbiology* 2007; 73(5):1630–1634.

10. Brandt M, Brown C, Burkhart J, Burton N, Cox-Ganser J, Damon S, et al. Mold Prevention Strategies and Possible Health Effects in the Aftermath of Hurricanes and Major Floods. *MMWR Recommendations and Reports* 2006; 55(RR-8):1–27.

11. Goddard Institute for Space Studies. NASA Looks at Sea Level Rise, Hurricane Risks to New York City. 2007; Available at: http://www.giss.nasa.gov/research/news/20061024/ Accessed 01/27/2008.

12. Passy C. The Search for Sand is No Day at the Beach. *The New York Times;* September 16, 2007.

13. The H. John Heinz III Center for Science, Economics and the Environment. Evaluation of Erosion Hazards Summary. 2000; Prepared for the Federal Emergency Management Agency, Contract EMW-97-CO-0375:19.

14. Hansen JE. Scientific Reticence and Sea Level Rise. *Environmental Research Letters* 2007; 2.

15. United States Geological Survey. Wetlands Break Waves, Quell Surge Coastal Landscape Battles Weather to Protect Mainland. 2006; Available at: http://www.lacoast.gov/WATERMARKS/2006-03/2protectMainland/ USGS National Wetlands Research Center. Accessed 01/28/2008.

16. D'Amato G, Liccardi G, Frenguelli G. Thunderstorm-asthma and Pollen Allergy. *Allergy* 2007; 62(1):11–16.

17. National Climatic Data Center. Climate of 2005: Summary of Hurricane Katrina. 2005; Available at: http://www.ncdc.noaa.gov/oa/climate/research/2005/katrina.html NOAA Satellite and Information Service. Accessed 1/1/2008.

18. Institute on Climate and Planets. Climate Impacts in New York City: Sea Level Rise and Coastal Floods. 2004; Available at: http://icp.giss.nasa.gov/research/ppa/2002/impacts/introduction.html Goddard Institute for Space Studies, NASA. Accessed 01/27/2008.

19. Eaton L. New Orleans Recovery Is Slowed by Closed Hospitals. *The New York Times;* July 24, 2007.

20. Kessler RC, Hurricane Katrina Community Advisory Group. Hurricane Katrina's Impact on the Care of Survivors with Chronic Medical Conditions. *Journal of General Internal Medicine* 2007; 22(9):1225–1230.

21. Abramson D, Garfield R, Redlener I. The Recovery Divide: Poverty and the Widening Gap among Mississippi Children and Families Affected by

Hurricane Katrina. Columbia University, Mailman School of Public Health, 2007.

22. Mills E. Insurance in a Climate of Change. *Science* 2005; 309:1040–1044.

23. Associated Press. Allstate Will Not Insure Md. Coast; Won't Sell New Homeowner Policies in Parts of County. *The Capital*; 12/21/2006.

24. Dasgupta S, Laplante B, Meisner C, Wheeler D, Yan J. The Impact of Sea Level Rise on Developing Countries: A Comparative Analysis. World Bank Policy Research Working Paper 2007; 4136:1–51.

25. Glass TA, McAtee MJ. Behavioral Science at the Crossroads in Public Health: Extending Horizons, Envisioning the Future. *Social Science & Medicine*, 2006; 62(7):1650–1671.

26. Abbott C. *An Uncertain Future: Law Enforcement, National Security, and Climate Change.* London: Oxford Research Group; 2008.

27. Galea S, Brewin CR, Gruber M, Jones RT, King DW, King LA, et al. Exposure to Hurricane-Related Stressors and Mental Illness after Hurricane Katrina. *Archives of General Psychiatry* 2007; 64(12):1427–1434.

28. Gittelman M. Disasters and Psychosocial Rehabilitation: The Nature, Frequency, and Effects of Disasters. *International Journal of Mental Health* 2004; 32(4):51–69.

29. Morrissey SA, Reser JP. Natural Disasters, Climate Change and Mental Health Considerations for Rural Australia. *Australia Journal of Rural Health* 2007; 15(2):120–125.

30. Bourque LB, Siegel JM, Kano M, Wood MM. Weathering the Storm: The Impact of Hurricanes on Physical and Mental Health. *Annals of the American Academy of Political and Social Science* 2006; 604:129–150.

31. Kessler RC, Galea S, Gruber MJ, Sampson NA, Ursano RJ, Wessely S. Trends in Mental Illness and Suicidality after Hurricane Katrina. *Molecular Psychiatry* 2008; 13:374–384.

32. Weisler RH, Barbee JG, Townsend MH. Mental Health and Recovery in the Gulf Coast after Hurricanes Katrina and Rita. *Journal of the American Medical Association* 2006; 296(5):585–588.

33. Kohn R, Levav I, Garcia ID, Machuca ME, Tamashiro R. Prevalence, Risk Factors and Aging Vulnerability for Psychopathology Following a Natural Disaster in a Developing Country. *International Journal of Geriatric Psychiatry* 2005; 20(9):835–841.

34. Weems CF, Pina AA, Costa NM, Watts SE, Taylor LK, Cannon MF. Predisaster Trait Anxiety and Negative Affect Predict Posttraumatic Stress in Youths After Hurricane Katrina. *Journal of Consulting and Clinical Psychology* 2007; 75(1):154–159.

35. Kessler RC, Galea S, Jones RT, Parker HA. Hurricane Katrina Community Advisory Group. Mental Illness and Suicidality after Hurricane Katrina. *Bulletin of the World Health Organization* 2006; 84(12):930–939.

36. Doherty GW. Crises in Rural America: Critical Incidents, Trauma and Disasters. *Traumatology* 2004; 10(3):145–164.

37. Evans LG, Oehler-Stinnett J. Structure and Prevalence of PTSD Symptomatology in Children Who Have Experienced a Severe Tornado. *Psychology in the Schools* 2006; 43(3):283–295.

38. Miller TW, Kraus RF. Natural and Environmental Disasters: Psychological Issues and Clinical Responses. *Integrative Psychiatry* 1994; 10(3):128–132.

39. Brodie M, Weltzien E, Altman D, Blendon RJ, Benson JM. Experiences of Hurricane Katrina Evacuees in Houston Shelters: Implications for Future Planning. *American Journal of Public Health* 2006; 96(5):1402–1408.

40. Tarhule A. Damaging Rainfall and Flooding: The Other Sahel Hazards. *Climatic Change* 2005; 72:355–377.

41. Napier JL, Mandisodza AN, Andersen SM, Jost JT. System Justification in Responding to the Poor and Displaced in the Aftermath of Hurricane Katrina. *Analyses of Social Issues and Public Policy (ASAP)* 2006; 6(1):57–73.

42. IPCC, 2007: Summary for Policymakers. In: Solomon S, Qin D, Manning M, Chen Z, Marquis M, Averyt KB, et al, editors. *Climate Change 2007: The Physical Science Basis. Contribution of Working Group I to the Fourth Assessment Report of the Intergovernmental Panel on Climate Change.* Cambridge, United Kingdom, and New York: Cambridge University Press; 2007.

43. Solomon S, Qin D, Manning M, Alley RB, Berntsen T, Bindoff NL, et al. *Technical Summary.* In: Solomon S, Qin D, Manning M, Chen Z, Marquis M, Averyt KB, et al., editors. *Climate Change 2007: The Physical Science Basis. Contribution of Working Group I to the Fourth Assessment Report of the Intergovernmental Panel on Climate Change.* Cambridge, United Kingdom, and New York: Cambridge University Press; 2007.

44. Magrin G, García CG, Choque DC, Giménez JC, Moreno AR, Nagy GJ, et al. 2007: Latin America. In: Parry ML, Canziani OF, Palutikof JP, van der Linden, P.J., Hanson CE, editors. *Climate Change 2007: Impacts, Adaptation and Vulnerability. Contribution of Working Group II to the Fourth Assessment Report of the Intergovernmental Panel on Climate Change.* Cambridge, United Kingdom: Cambridge University Press; 2007, pp. 581–615.

45. Meier MF, Dyurgerov MB, Rick UK, O'Neel S, Pfeffer WT, Anderson RS, et al. Glaciers Dominate Eustatic Sea-Level Rise in the 21st Century. *Science* 2007; 317(5841):1064–1067.

46. Brown P. Melting Ice Cap Triggering Earthquakes. *Guardian Unlimited*; September 8, 2007.

47. NASA Earth Observatory. Greenland Melt Accelerating, According to CU-Boulder Study. 2007; Available at: http://earthobservatory.nasa.gov/Newsroom/MediaAlerts/2007/2007121126008.html Accessed 1/4/2008.

48. National Snow and Ice Data Center. Frequently Asked Questions about Sea Ice. 2006; Available at: http://nsidc.org/news/press/2007_seaiceminimum/20070810_faq.html University of Colorado. Accessed 01/27/2008.

49. National Snow and Ice Data Center. Arctic Sea Ice Shatters All Previous Record Lows. 2007; Available at: http://nsidc.org/news/press/2007_seaiceminimum/20071001_pressrelease.html University of Colorado. Accessed 01/27/2008.

50. Rignot E, Bamber JL, Van Den Broeke, Michiel R., Davis C, et al. Recent Antarctic Ice Mass Loss from Radar Interferometry and Regional Climate Modeling. *Nature Geoscience* 2008; 1(2): 106–110.

51. Overpeck JT, Otto-Bliesner BL, Miller GH, Muhs DR, Alley RB, Kiehl JT. Paleoclimatic Evidence for Future Ice-Sheet Instability and Rapid Sea-Level Rise. *Science* 2006; 311(5768):1747–1750.

52. Pew Center on Global Climate Change. Hurricanes and Global Warming—Q&A. 2007; Available at: http://www.pewclimate.org/hurricanes.cfm#2007 Pew Center on Global Climate Change. Accessed 01/28/2008.

53. Michaels PJ, Knappenberger PC, Davis RE. Sea-surface Temperatures and Tropical Cyclones in the Atlantic Basin. *Geophysical Research Letters* 2006; 33:doi:10.1029/2006GL025757.

54. Trenberth KE, Shea DJ. Atlantic Hurricanes and Natural Variability in 2005. *Geophysical Research Letters* 2006; 33:doi:10.1029/2006GL026894.

55. Pielke J, RA, Landsea C, Mayfield M, Laver J, Pasch R. Hurricanes and Global Warming. *Bulletin of the American Meteorological Society* 2005; 86(11):1571–1575.

56. Webster PJ, Holland GJ, Curry JA, Chang HR. Changes in Tropical Cyclone Number, Duration, and Intensity in a Warming Environment. *Science* 2005; 309:1844–1846.

57. Emanuel K. Increasing Destructiveness of Tropical Cyclones over the Past 30 Years. *Nature* 2005; 436:686–688.

58. Kossin JP, Vimont DJ. A More General Framework for Understanding Atlantic Hurricane Variability and Trends. *Bulletin of the American Meteorological Society* 2007; 88:1767–1781.

59. Knupp KR, Walters J, Biggerstaff M. Doppler Profiler and Radar Observations of Boundary Layer Variability during the Landfall of Tropical Storm Gabrielle. *Journal of Atmospheric Sciences* 2006; 63:234–251.

## CHAPTER 7

1. Patz JA, Lindsay SW. New Challenges, New Tools: The Impact of Climate Change on Infectious Diseases. *Current Opinions in Microbiology* 1999; 2(4):445–451.

2. Vittor AY, Gilman RH, Tielsch J, Glass G, Shields T, Lozano WS, et al. The Effect of Deforestation on the Human-Biting Rate of *Anopheles darlingi*, the Primary Vector of Falciparum Malaria in the Peruvian Amazon. *American Journal of Tropical Medicine and Hygiene* 2006; 74(1):3–11.

3. Roberts JR, Reigart JR. Does Anything Beat DEET? *Pediatric Annals* 2004; 33(7):444–453.

4. Morens DM, Fauci AS. Dengue and Hemorrhagic Fever: A Potential Threat to Public Health in the United States. *Journal of the American Medical Association* 2008; 299(2):214–216.

5. Hales S, de Wet N, Maindonald J, Woodward A. Potential Effect of Population and Climate Changes on Global Distribution of Dengue Fever: An Empirical Model. *The Lancet* 2002; 360(9336):830–834.

6. Epstein PR. West Nile Virus and the Climate. *Journal of Urban Health* 2001; 78(2):367–371.

7. Division of Vector Borne Infectious Diseases, National Center for Zoonotic, Vector-Borne, and Enteric Diseases. 2007 West Nile Virus Activity in the United States, Reported to CDC as of November 13, 2007. Available at: http://www.cdc.gov/ncidod/dvbid/westnile/surv&controlCaseCount07_detailed. htm Centers for Disease Control and Prevention. Accessed 11/18/2007.

8. Patz JA, Reisen WK. Immunology, Climate Change and Vector-Borne Diseases. *Trends in Immunology* 2001; 22(4):171–172.

9. Stenseth NC, Samia NI, Viljugrein H, Kausrud KL, Begon M, Davis S, et al. Plague Dynamics are Driven by Climate Variation. *Proceedings of the National Academy of Sciences* 2006; 103(35):13110–13115.

10. Parmenter RR, Yadav EP, Parmenter CA, Ettestad P, Gage KL. Incidence of Plague Associated with Increased Winter-Spring Precipitation in New Mexico. *American Journal of Tropical Medicine Hygiene* 1999; 61(5):814–821.

11. Lindgren E, Gustafson R. Tick-Borne Encephalitis in Sweden and Climate Change. *The Lancet* 2001; 358:16–18.

12. Glass GE, Cheek JE, Patz JA, Shields TM, Doyle TJ, Thoroughman DA, et al. Using Remotely Sensed Data to Identify Areas at Risk for Hantavirus Pulmonary Syndrome. *Emerging Infectious Diseases* 2000; 6(3):238–247.

13. Weiss RA, McMichael AJ. Social and Environmental Risk Factors in the Emergence of Infectious Diseases. *Nature Medicine Supplement* 2004; 10(12):S70–S76.

14. Epidemic and Pandemic Alert and Response. Summary of Probable SARS Cases with Onset of Illness from 1 November 2002 to 31 July 2003. 2004; Available at: http://www.who.int/csr/sars/country/table2004_04_21/en/index.html World Health Organization. Accessed 01/08/2008.

15. Colwell RR, Patz JA. Climate, Infectious Disease and Health: An Interdisciplinary Perspective. 1998. Report to the American Academy of Microbiology, Washington, DC.

16. McLaughlin JB, DePaola A, Bopp CA, Martinek KA, Napolilli NP, Allison CG, et al. Outbreak of Vibrio Parahaemolyticus Gastroenteritis Associated with Alaskan Oysters. *New England Journal of Medicine* 2005; 353(14):1463–1470.

17. Arizona Department of Health Services. Arizona Valley Fever Report: December 2007. 2007; Available at: http://azdhs.gov/phs/oids/epi/disease/cocci/ cocci_report_dec_2007.pdf Accessed 01/19/2008.

18. Kovats RS, Edwards SJ, Hajat S, Armstrong BG, Ebi KLB. The Effect of Temperature on Food Poisoning: A Time-series Analysis of Salmonellosis in Ten European Countries. *Epidemiology and Infection* 2004; 132:443–453.

19. Louis VR, Gillespie IA, O'Brien SJ, Russek-Cohen E, Pearson AD, Colwell RR. Temperature-Driven Campylobacter Seasonality in England and Wales. *Applied Environmental Microbiology* 2005; 71(1):85–92.

20. Ko C, Yen C, Yen J, Yang M. Psychosocial Impact Among the Public of the Severe Acute Respiratory Syndrome Epidemic in Taiwan. *Psychiatry and Clinical Neurosciences* 2006; 60(4):397–403.

21. Lee TMC, Chi I, Chung LWM, Chou K. Ageing and Psychological Response during the Post-SARS Period. *Aging & Mental Health* 2006; 10(3):303–311.

22. Lee AM, Wong JGWS, McAlonan GM, Cheung V, Cheung C, Sham PC, et al. Stress and Psychological Distress Among SARS Survivors 1 Year after the Outbreak. *The Canadian Journal of Psychiatry* 2007; 52(4):233–240.

23. Nagao K, Okuno M, Shindou E. Mental Symptoms Induced by a Massive Outbreak of Infectious Disease (Enterhemorragic Escherichia Coli 0157) in Elementary School Children: II. Six Cases of Delayed and Reactivated Stress-Related Disorders, Including PTSD. *Japanese Journal of Child and Adolescent Psychiatry* 2001; 42(4):315–322.

24. Boivin MJ. Effects of Early Cerebral Malaria on Cognitive Ability in Senegalese Children. *Journal of Developmental & Behavioral Pediatrics* 2002; 23(5):353–364.

25. Carter JA, Murira GM, Ross AJ, Mung'ala-Odera V, Newton CRJC. Speech and Language Sequelae of Severe Malaria in Kenyan Children. *Brain Injury* 2003; 17(3):217–224.

26. Carter JA, Mung'ala-Odera V, Neville BGR, Murira G, Mturi N, Musumba C, et al. Persistent Neurocognitive Impairments Associated with Severe Falciparum Malaria in Kenyan Children. *Journal of Neurology, Neurosurgery & Psychiatry* 2005; 76(4):476–481.

27. Olness K. Effects on Brain Development Leading to Cognitive Impairement: A Worldwide Epidemic. *Journal of Developmental & Behavioral Pediatrics* 2003; 24(2):120–130.

28. Pancharoen C, Thisyakorn U. Neurological Manifestations in Dengue Patients. *Southeast Asian Journal of Tropical Medicine and Public Health* 2001; 32(2):341–345.

29. Haaland KY, Sadek J, Pergam S, Echevarria LA, Davis LE, Goade D, et al. Mental Status after West Nile Virus Infection. *Emerging Infectious Diseases* 2006; 12(8):1260–1262.

30. Sanchez SH, Katz CL. International Disaster Mental Health Services: A Survey. *Psychiatric Services* 2006; 57(3):420–421.

31. American Academy of Pediatrics Committee on Environmental Health. West Nile Virus Information: Follow Safety Precautions When Using DEET on Children. 2003; Available at: http://www.aap.org/family/wnv-jun03.htm American Academy of Pediatrics. Accessed 01/19/2008.

32. Division of Vector-Borne Infectious Diseases. Updated Information Regarding Mosquito Repellents. 2006; Available at: http://www.cdc.gov/

ncidod/dvbid/westnile/RepellentUpdates.htm Centers for Disease Control and Prevention. Accessed 01/19/2008.

33. Kuhn K, Campbell-Lendrum D, Haines A, Cox J. Using Climate to Predict Infectious Disease Epidemics. World Health Organization, Geneva, 2005.

## CHAPTER 8

1. Gould E. Manager's Report to the Board of Directors, Federal Crop Insurance Corporation. Report No. 2906. 2007. U.S. Department of Agriculture, Washington, DC.

2. Pirog R. Checking the Food Odometer: Comparing Food Miles for Local Versus Conventional Produce Sales to Iowa Institutions. Leopold Center for Sustainable Agriculture, Iowa State University. Ames, IA, 2003.

3. Long SP, Ainsworth EA, Leakey, Andrew D. B., Nosberger J, Ort DR. Food for Thought: Lower-Than-Expected Crop Yield Stimulation with Rising $CO_2$ Concentrations. *Science* 2006; 312:1918–1921.

4. Lobell DB, Field CB. Global Scale Climate-Crop Yield Relationships and the Impacts of Recent Warming. *Environmental Research Letters* 2007; 2(014002): November 22, 2007.

5. Frumhoff PC, McCarthy JJ, Melillo JM, Moser SC, Wuebbles DJ. Confronting Climate Change in the U.S. Northeast: Science, Impacts, and Solutions. 2007; Synthesis Report of the Northeast Climate Impacts Assessment (NECIA), Union of Concerned Scientists. Washington, DC.

6. Wohlsen M. California Citrus Growers Face Big Losses as Cold Snap Continues. SFGate.com 1/14/2007.

7. Harrington R, Fleming RA, Woiwod IP. Climate Change Impacts on Insect Management and Conservation in Temperate Regions: Can They Be Predicted? *Agricultural and Forest Entomology* 2001; 3:233–240.

8. Cannon, Raymond J. C. The Implications of Predicted Climate Change for Insect Pests in the UK, with Emphasis on Non-indigenous Species. *Global Change Biology* 1998; 4:785–796.

9. Chen C, McCarl BA. An Investigation of the Relationship between Pesticide Usage and Climate Change. *Climatic Change* 2001; 50:475–487.

10. Brown TP, Rumsby PC, Capleton AC, Rushton L, Levy LS. Pesticides and Parkinson's Disease—Is There a Link? *Environmental Health Perspectives* 2006; 114:156–164.

11. Roberts EM, English PB, Grether JK, Windham GC, Somberg L, Wolff C. Maternal Residence Near Agricultural Pesticide Applications and Autism Spectrum Disorders among Children in the California Central Valley. *Environmental Health Perspectives* 2007; 115(10):1482–1489.

12. Brent RL, Weitzman M. The Current State of Knowledge About the Effects, Risks, and Science of Children's Environmental Exposures. *Pediatrics* 2004; 113(4):1158–1166.

13. Pimentel D, Harvey C, Resosudarmo P, Sinclair K, Kurz D, McNair M, et al. Environmental and Economic Costs of Soil Erosion and Conservation Benefits. *Science* 1995; 267:1117–1122.

14. Sitch S, Cox PM, Collings WJ, Huntingford C. Indirect Radiative Forcing of Climate Change through Ozone Effects on the Land-Carbon Sink. *Nature* 2007; 48:791–795.

15. Key N, Roberts MJ. Measures of Trends in Farm Size Tell Differing Stories. *Amber Waves* 2007; 5(5): Statistics. A newsletter of United States Department of Agriculture, Economic Research Service, Washington, DC.

16. Andersson K, Ohlsson T, Olsson P. Screening Life Cycle Assessment (LCA) of Tomato Ketchup: A Case Study. *Journal of Cleaner Production* 1998; 6(3–4):277–288.

17. USDA Economic Research Service. Food CPI, Prices and Expenditures: Food Expenditures by Families and Individuals as a Share of Disposable Personal Money Income. 2007; United States Department of Agriculture.

18. Funes F, Garcia L, Bourque M, Perez N, Rosset P. *Sustainable Agriculture and Resistance: Transforming Food Production in Cuba.* Oakland, CA: Food First Books; 2001.

19. Behrenfeld MJ, O'Malley RT, Siegel DA, McClain CR, Sarmiento JL, Feldman GC, et al. Climate-Driven Trends in Contemporary Ocean Productivity. *Nature* 2006; 444:752–755.

20. Doney SC. Plankton in a Warmer World. *Nature* 2006; 444:695–696.

21. Ruttimann J. Sick Seas. *Nature* 2006; 442:978–980.

22. Naylor RL, Goldburg RJ, Primavera JH, Kautsky N, Beveridge, Malcolm C. M., Clay J, et al. Effect of Aquaculture on World Fish Supplies. *Nature* 2000; 405:1017–1024.

23. Aschner M, Syversen T. Methylmercury: Recent Advances in the Understanding of Its Neurotoxicity. *Therapeutic Drug Monitoring* 2005; 27:278–283.

24. Turetsky MR, Harden JW, Friedli HR, Flannigan M, Payne N, Crock J, et al. Wildfires Threaten Mercury Stocks in Northern Soils. *Geophysical Research Letters* 2006; 33:doi:10:1029/2005GL025595.

25. Knobeloch L, Gliori G, Anderson H. Assessment of Methylmercury Exposure in Wisconsin. *Environmental Research* 2007; 103(2):205–210.

26. Cline WR. *Global Warming and Climate Change: Impact Assessments by Country.* Washington, DC: Center for Global Development and Peterson Institute for International Economics; 2007.

27. Steinfeld H, Gerber P, Wassenaar T, Castel V, Rosales M, de Haan C. Livestock's Long Shadow: Environmental Issues and Options. 2006. Food and Agricultural Organization, United Nations, New York.

28. McMichael AJ, Powles JW, Butler CD, Uauy R. Food, Livestock Production, Energy, Climate Change, and Health. *The Lancet* 2007; 370(9594):1253–1263.

29. Shapouri H, Duffield JA, Wang M. The Energy Balance of Corn Ethanol: An Update. 2002; Agricultural Economic Report No. 814. U.S. Department of

Agriculture, Office of the Chief Economist, Office of Energy Policy and New Uses, Washington, DC.

30. Farrell AE, Plevin RJ, Turner BT, Jones AD, O'Hare M, Kammen DM. Ethanol Can Contribute to Energy and Environmental Goals. *Science* 2006; 311(5760):506–508.

31. Righelato R, Spracklen DV. Environment: Carbon Mitigation by Biofuels or by Saving and Restoring Forests? *Science* 2007; 317(5840):902.

32. Scharlemann JPW, Laurance WF. How Green Are Biofuels? *Science* 2008; 319:43–44.

33. Tanner EM, Finn-Stevenson M. Nutrition and Brain Development: Social Policy Implications. *American Journal of Orthopsychiatry* 2002; 72(2):182–193.

34. Wachs TD. Nutritional Deficits and Behavioural Development. *International Journal of Behavioral Development* 2000; 24(4):435–441.

35. Lee Y, Lee MK, Chun KH, Lee YK, Yoon SJ. Trauma Experience of North Korean Refugees in China. *American Journal of Preventive Medicine* 2001; 20(3):225–229.

36. Yu S, Hannum E. Food for Thought: Poverty, Family Nutritional Environment, and Children's Educational Performance in Rural China. *Sociological Perspectives* 2007; 50(1):53–77.

37. Bohle HG, Downing TE, Watts MJ. Climate Change and Social Vulnerability: Toward a Sociology and Geography of Food Insecurity. *Global Environmental Change* 1994; 4(1):37–48.

38. Chilton M, Booth S. Hunger of the Body and Hunger of the Mind: African American Women's Perceptions of Food Insecurity, Health and Violence. *Journal of Nutrition Education and Behavior* 2007; 39(3):116–125.

39. Cohen M. Environmental Toxins and Health: The Health Impact of Pesticides. *Australian Family Physician* 2007; 36(12):1002–1004.

40. Eskenazi B, Marks AR, Bradman A, Harley K, Barr DB, Johnson C, et al. Organophosphate Pesticide Exposure and Neurodevelopment in Young Mexican-American Children. *Environmental Health Perspectives* 2007; 115(5):792–798.

41. Sanchez Lizardi P, O'Rourke MK, Morris RJ. The Effects of Organophosphate Pesticide Exposure on Hispanic Children's Cognitive and Behavioral Functioning. *Journal of Pediatric Psychology* 2008; 33(1):91–101.

## CHAPTER 9

1. Morgan JA, Milchunas DG, LeCain DR, West M, Mosier AR. Carbon Dioxide Enrichment Alters Plant Community Structure and Accelerates Shrub Growth in the Shortgrass Steppe. *Proceedings of the National Academy of Sciences* 2007; 104(37):14724–14729.

2. Johnson WC, Millett BV, Gilmanov T, Voldseth RA, Guntenspergen GR, Naugle DE. Vulnerability of Northern Prairie Wetlands to Climate Change. *BioScience* 2005; 55(10):863–872.

3. Schwandt JW. Whitebark Pine in Peril: A Case for Restoration. 2006. A Report to USDA Forest Service, Forest Health Protection. Coeur d'Alene, ID.

4. Chambers JQ, Fisher JI, Zeng H, Chapman EL, Baker DB, Hurtt GC. Hurricane Katrina's Carbon Footprint on U.S. Gulf Coast Forests. *Science* 2007; 318:1107.

5. Worm B, Barbier EB, Beaumont N, Duffy JE, Folke C, Halpern BS, et al. Impacts of Biodiversity Loss on Ocean Ecosystem Services. *Science* 2006; 314:787–790.

6. Louisiana Universities Marine Consortium. Dead Zone Size Near Top End. 7/28/2007. Louisiana State University, Baton Rouge, LA

7. Service RF. "Dead Zone" Reappears Off Oregon Coast. *Science NOW Daily News* 7/31/2007.

8. LoGiudice K, Ostfeld RS, Schmidt KA, Keesing F. The Ecology of Infectious Disease: Effects of Host Diversity and Community Composition on Lyme Disease Risk. *Proceedings of the National Academy of Sciences* 2003; 100(2):567–571.

9. Chapin, F. Stuart III, Zavaleta ES, Eviner VT, Naylor RL, Vitousek PM, et al. Consequences of Changing Biodiversity. *Nature* 2000; 405:234–242.

10. Stern N. The Stern Review Report on the Economics of Climate Change. 2006. Available at: http://www.hm-treasury.gov.uk/independent_reviews/stern_review_economics_climate_change/stern_review_report.cfm Accessed 1/31/2008.

11. Knorr W, Gobron N, Scholze M, Kaminski T, Schnur R, Pinty B. Impact of Terrestrial Biosphere Carbon Exchanges on the Anomalous $CO_2$ Increase in 2002–2003. *Geophysical Research Letters* 2007; 34(L09703).

12. Paulson A. In Coal Country, Heat Rises over Latest Method of Mining. *Christian Science Monitor*; January 3, 2006.

13. Kutscher CF, editor. *Tackling Climate Change in the U.S.: Potential Carbon Emissions Reductions from Energy Efficiency and Renewable Energy by 2030.* Boulder, CO: American Solar Energy Society; 2007.

14. Wigley TML. A Combined Mitigation/Geoengineering Approach to Climate Stabilization. *Science* 2006; 314:452–454.

15. Brewer PG. Evaluating a Technological Fix for Climate. *Proceedings of the National Academy of Sciences* 2007; 104(24):9915–9916.

16. Barnaby F, Kemp J, editors. *Secure Energy? Civil Nuclear Power, Security and Global Warming.* London, United Kingdom: Oxford Research Group; 2007.

17. Bunker DE, Declerck F, Bradford JC, Colwell RK, Perfecto I, Phillips OL, et al. Species Loss and Aboveground Carbon Storage in a Tropical Forest. *Science* 2005; 310(5750):1029–1031.

## CHAPTER 10

1. Vlek C, Steg L. Human Behavior and Environmental Sustainability: Problems, Driving Forces, and Research Topics. *Journal of Social Issues* 2007; 63(1):1–19.

2. Barr S, Gilg A, Shaw G. Promoting Sustainable Lifestyles: A Social Marketing Approach. University of Exeter. 2006.

3. Kaiser FG, Fuhrer U. Ecological Behavior's Dependency on Different Forms of Knowledge. *Applied Psychology: An International Review* 2003; 52(4):598–613.

4. Gatersleben B, Steg L, Vlek C. Measurement and Determinants of Environmentally Significant Consumer Behavior. *Environment and Behavior* 2002; 34(3):335–362.

5. Halpern F, Bates C, Beales G, Heathfield A. Personal Responsibility and Changing Behaviour: The State of Knowledge and Its Implications for Public Policy. London: Cabinet Office: Prime Minister's Strategy Unit. 2004.

6. Vlek C. Essential Psychology for Environmental Policy Making. *International Journal of Psychology* 2000; 35(2):153–167.

7. Dahlstrand U, Biel A. Pro-Environmental Habits: Propensity Levels in Behavioral Change. *Journal of Applied Social Psychology* 1997; 27(7):588–601.

8. Hanna FJ. *Therapy with Difficult Clients: Using the Precursors Model to Awaken Change.* Washington, DC: American Psychological Association; 2002.

9. Lorenzoni I, Pidgeon NF. Public Views on Climate Change: European and USA Perspectives. *Climatic Change* 2006; 77:73–95.

10. Osbaldiston R. 2005. Meta-Analysis of the Responsible Environmental Behavior Literature. PhD diss., University of Missouri, Columbia.

11. Weber EU. Experience-Based and Description-Based Perceptions of Long-Term Risk: Why Global Warming Does Not Scare Us (Yet). *Climatic Change* 2006; 77:103–120.

12. Stern PC. Psychology and the Science of Human-Environment Interactions. *American Psychologist* 2000; 55(5):523–530.

13. Bamberg S, Möser G. Twenty Years after Hines, Hungerford, and Tomera: A New Meta-Analysis of Psycho-Social Determinants of Pro-Environmental Behaviour. *Journal of Environmental Psychology* 2007; 27(1):14–25.

14. Kaiser FG, Wölfing S, Fuhrer U. Environmental Attitude and Ecological Behaviour. *Journal of Environmental Psychology* 1999; 19(1):1–19.

15. Kilbourne WE, Beckmann SC, Lewis A, Van Dam Y. A Multinational Examination of the Role of the Dominant Social Paradigm in Environmental Attitudes of University Students. *Environment and Behavior* 2001; 33(2):209–228.

16. Rauwald KS, Moore CF. Environmental Attitudes as Predictors of Policy Support across Three Countries. *Environment and Behavior* 2002; 34(6):709–739.

17. Sterman JD, Sweeney LB. Understanding Public Complacency about Climate Change: Adults' Mental Models of Climate Change Violate Conservation of Matter. *Climatic Change* 2007; 80:213–238.

18. Jamieson D. An American Paradox. *Climatic Change* 2006; 77:97–102.

19. Bazerman MH. Climate Change as a Predictable Surprise. *Climatic Change* 2006; 77:179–193.

20. Oskamp S. Psychological Contributions to Achieving an Ecologically Sustainable Future for Humanity. *Journal of Social Issues* 2000; 56(3):373–390.

21. Oskamp S. Environmentally Responsible Behavior: Teaching and Promoting It Effectively. *Analyses of Social Issues and Public Policy* 2002; 2(1):173–182.

22. Clark CF, Kotchen MJ, Moore MR. Internal and External Influences on Pro-Environmental Behavior: Participation in a Green Electricity Program. *Journal of Environmental Psychology* 2003; 23:237–246.

23. Heath Y, Gifford R. Free-Market Ideology and Environmental Degradation: The Case of Belief in Global Climate Change. *Environment and Behavior* 2006; 38(1):48–71.

24. Rachlinski JJ. The Psychology of Global Climate Change. *University of Illinois Law Review* 2000; (1):299–319.

25. Belzer RB. Discounting Across Generations: Necessary, Not Suspect. *Risk Analysis* 2000; 20(6):779–792.

26. Hatfield J, Job RFS. Optimism Bias about Environmental Degradation: The Role of the Range of Impact of Precautions. *Journal of Environmental Psychology* 2001; 21(1):17–30.

27. Pahl S, Harris PR, Todd HA, Rutter DR. Comparative Optimism for Environmental Risks. *Journal of Environmental Psychology* 2005; 25(1):1–11.

28. Sunstein CR. The Availability Heuristic, Intuitive Cost-Benefit Analysis, and Climate Change. *Climatic Change* 2006; 77:195–210.

29. Dyson T. On Development, Demography and Climate Change: The End of the World As We Know It? *Population and Environment: A Journal of Interdisciplinary Studies* 2005; 27(2):117–149.

30. Norgaard KM. "We Don't Really Want to Know": Environmental Justice and Socially Organized Denial of Global Warming in Norway. *Organization & Environment* 2006; 19(3):347–370.

31. Stoll-Kleemann S, O'Riordan T, Jaeger CC. The Psychology of Denial Concerning Climate Mitigation Measures: Evidence from Swiss Focus Groups. *Global Environmental Change* 2001; 11:107–117.

32. Leiserowitz A. Climate Change Risk Perception and Policy Preferences: The Role of Affect, Imagery, and Values. *Climatic Change* 2006; 77:45–72.

33. Fransson N, Gärling T. Environmental Concern: Conceptual Definitions, Measurement Methods, and Research Findings. *Journal of Environmental Psychology* 1999; 19(4):369–382.

34. Thogersen J, Ölander F. To What Degree Are Environmentally Beneficial Choices Reflective of a General Conservation Stance? *Environment and Behavior* 2006; 38(4):550–569.

35. Brossard D, Shanahan J, McComas K. Are Issue-Cycles Culturally Constructed? A Comparison of French and American Coverage of Global Climate Change. *Mass Communication and Society* 2004; 7(3):359–377.

36. Schultz PW. The Structure of Environmental Concern: Concern for Self, Other People, and the Biosphere. *Journal of Environmental Psychology* 2001; 21(4):327–339.

37. Diekmann A, Franzen A. The Wealth of Nations and Environmental Concern. *Environment and Behavior* 1999; 31(4):540–549.

38. Franzen A. Environmental Attitudes in International Comparison: An Analysis of the ISSP Surveys 1993 and 2000. *Social Science Quarterly* 2003; 84(2):297–308.

39. Krosnick JA, Holbrook AL, Lowe L, Visser PS. The Origins and Consequences of Democratic Citizens' Policy Agendas: A Study of Popular Concerns about Global Warming. *Climatic Change* 2006; 77:7–43.

40. Baron J. Thinking about Global Warming. *Climatic Change* 2006; 77:137–150.

41. Kurz T, Donaghue N, Rapley M, Walker I. The Ways that People Talk about Natural Resources: Discursive Strategies as Barriers to Environmentally Sustainable Practices. *British Journal of Social Psychology* 2005; 44(4):603–620.

42. Berenguer J. The Effect of Empathy in Proenvironmental Attitudes and Behaviors. *Environment and Behavior* 2007; 39(2):269–283.

43. Kals E, Schumacher D, Montada L. Emotional Affinity Toward Nature as a Motivational Basis to Protect Nature. *Environment and Behavior* 1999; 31(2):178–202.

44. Mitchell MM, Brown KM, Morris-Villagran M, Villagran PD. The Effects of Anger, Sadness and Happiness on Persuasive Message Processing: A Test of the Negative State Relief Model. *Communication Monographs* 2001; 68(4):347–359.

45. Sundblad E, Biel A, Gärling T. Cognitive and Affective Risk Judgments Related to Climate Change. *Journal of Environmental Psychology* 2007; 27:97–106.

46. Norgaard KM. "People Want to Protect Themselves a Little Bit": Emotions, Denial, and Social Movement Nonparticipation. *Sociological Inquiry* 2006; 76(3):372–396.

47. Bamberg S. How Does Environmental Concern Influence Specific Environmentally Related Behaviors? A New Answer to an Old Question. *Journal of Environmental Psychology* 2003; 23(1):21–32.

48. Schultz PW, Zelezny L. Values as Predictors of Environmental Attitudes: Evidence for Consistency Across 14 Countries. *Journal of Environmental Psychology* 1999; 19(3):255–265.

49. Hernández B, Suárez E, Martínez-Torvisco J, Hess S. The Study of Environmental Beliefs by Facet Analysis: Research in the Canary Islands, Spain. *Environment and Behavior* 2000; 32(5):612–636.

50. Nordlund AM, Garvill J. Value Structures Behind Proenvironmental Behavior. *Environment and Behavior* 2002; 34(6):740–756.

51. Meinhold JL, Malkus AJ. Adolescent Environmental Behaviors: Can Knowledge, Attitudes, and Self-Efficacy Make a Difference? *Environment and Behavior* 2005; 37(4):511–532.

52. Nordlund AM, Garvill J. Effects of Values, Problem Awareness, and Personal Norm on Willingness to Reduce Personal Car Use. *Journal of Environmental Psychology* 2003; 23(4):339–347.

53. O'Connor RE, Bord RJ, Fisher A. Risk Perceptions, General Environmental Beliefs, and Willingness to Address Climate Change. *Risk Analysis* 1999; 19(3):461–471.

54. Eriksson L, Garvill J, Nordlund AM. Interrupting Habitual Car Use: The Importance of Car Habit Strength and Moral Motivation for Personal Car Use Reduction. *Transportation Research Part F: Traffic Psychology and Behaviour* 2008; 11(1):10–23.

55. Howard GS. Adapting Human Lifestyles for the 21st Century. *American Psychologist* 2000; 55(5):509–515.

56. Hodgkinson SP, Innes JM. The Prediction of Ecological and Environmental Belief Systems: The Differential Contributions of Social Conservatism and Beliefs about Money. *Journal of Environmental Psychology* 2000; 20:285–294.

57. Corraliza JA, Berenguer J. Environmental Values, Beliefs, and Actions: A Situational Approach. *Environment and Behavior* 2000; 32(6):832–848.

58. Witte K. *Fear As Motivator, Fear As Inhibitor: Using Extended Parallel Process to Explain Fear Appeal Successes and Failures*. In: Anderson PA, Guerrero LK, editors. *Handbook of Communication and Emotion: Research, Theory, Applications, and Contexts*. San Diego: Academic Press; 1998, pp. 423–450.

59. Costarelli S, Colloca P. The Effects of Attitudinal Ambivalence on Pro-Environmental Behavioural Intentions. *Journal of Environmental Psychology* 2004; 24(3):279–288.

60. Kuhn KM. Message Format and Audience Values: Interactive Effects of Uncertainty Information and Environmental Attitudes on Perceived Risk. *Journal of Environmental Psychology* 2000; 20(1):41–51.

61. Kaiser FG, Ranney M, Hartig T, Bowler PA. Ecological Behavior, Environmental Attitude, and Feelings of Responsibility for the Environment. *European Psychologist* 1999; 4(2):59–74.

62. Eiser JR, Reicher SD, Podpadec TJ. Global Changes and Local Accidents: Consistency in Attributions for Environmental Effects. *Journal of Applied Social Psychology* 1995; 25(17):1518–1529.

63. Uzzell DL. The Psycho-Spatial Dimension of Global Environmental Problems. *Journal of Environmental Psychology* 2000; 20:307–318.

64. Blake DE. Contextual Effects on Environmental Attitudes and Behavior. *Environment and Behavior* 2001; 33(5):708–725.

65. Devine-Wright P, Devine-Wright H, Fleming P. Situational Influences Upon Children's Beliefs about Global Warming and Energy. *Environmental Education Research* 2004; 10:493–506.

66. Gärling T, Fuijii S, Gärling A, Jakobsson C. Moderating Effects of Social Value Orientation on Determinants of Proenvironmental Behavior Intention. *Journal of Environmental Psychology* 2003; 23(1):1–9.

67. Dessai S, Adger WN, Hulme M, Turnpenny J, Kohler J, Warren R. Defining and Experiencing Dangerous Climate Change: An Editorial Essay. *Climatic Change* 2004; 64:11–25.

68. McDaniels T, Axelrod LJ, Slovic P. Characterizing Perception of Ecological Risk. *Risk Analysis* 1995; 15(5):575–588.

69. Viscusi WK, Zeckhauser RJ. The Perception and Valuation of the Risks of Climate Change: A Rational and Behavioral Blend. *Climatic Change* 2006; 77:151–177.

70. Grothmann T, Patt A. Adaptive Capacity and Human Cognition: The Process of Individual Adaptation to Climate Change. *Global Environmental Change* 2005; 15:199–213.

71. Arvai J, Bridge G, Dolsak N, Franzese R, Koontz T, Luginbuhl A, et al. Adaptive Management of the Global Climate Problem: Bridging the Gap between Climate Research and Climate Policy. *Climatic Change* 2006; 78:217–225.

72. Smit B, Wandel J. Adaptation, Adaptive Capacity, and Vulnerability. *Global Environmental Change* 2006; 16:282–292.

73. Tschakert P. Views from the Vulnerable: Understanding Climatic and Other Stressors in the Sahel. *Global Environmental Change* 2007; 17:381–396.

74. Lorenzoni I, Leiserowitz A, De Franca Doria M, Poortinga W, Pidgeon NF. Cross-National Comparisons of Image Associations with "Global Warming" and "Climate Change" Among Laypeople in the United States of America and Great Britain. *Journal of Risk Research* 2006; 9(3):265–281.

75. Donohoe M. Causes and Health Consequences of Environmental Degradation and Social Injustice. *Social Science & Medicine*, 2003; 56(3):573–587.

76. Kaiser FG, Shimoda TA. Responsibility as a Predictor of Ecological Behavior. *Journal of Environmental Psychology* 1999; 19(3):243–253.

77. O'Connor RE, Bord RJ, Yarnal B, Wiefek N. Who Wants to Reduce Greenhouse Gas Emissions? *Social Science Quarterly* 2002; 83(1):1–17.

78. Meijnders AL, Midden CJH, Wilke HAM. Communications about Environmental Risks and Risk-Reducing Behavior: The Impact of Fear on Information Processing. *Journal of Applied Social Psychology* 2001; 31:754–777.

79. Meijnders AL, Midden CJH, Wilke HAM. Role of Negative Emotions in Communication about $CO_2$ Risks. *Risk Analysis* 2001; 21(5):955–966.

80. García-Mira R, Real JE, Romay J. Temporal and Spatial Dimensions in the Perception of Environmental Problems: An Investigation of the Concept of Environmental Hyperopia. *International Journal of Psychology* 2005; 40(1):5–10.

81. Vaidyanathan R, Aggarwal P. Using Commitments to Drive Consistency: Enhancing the Effectiveness of Cause-related Marketing Communications. *Journal of Marketing Communications* 2005; 11:231–246.

82. Syme GJ, Kals E, Nancarrow BE, Montada L. Ecological Risks and Community Perceptions of Fairness and Justice: A Cross-Cultural Model. *Risk Analysis* 2000; 20(6):905–916.

83. Lazo JK, Kinnell JC, Fisher A. Expert and Layperson Perceptions of Ecosystem Risk. *Risk Analysis* 2000; 20(2):179–193.

84. Hersch J, Viscusi WK. The Generational Divide in Support for Environmental Policies: European Evidence. *Climatic Change* 2006; 77:121–136.

85. Nooney JG, Woodrum E, Hoban TJ, Clifford WB. Environmental Worldview and Behavior: Consequences of Dimensionality in a Survey of North Carolinians. *Environment and Behavior* 2003; 35:763–783.

86. Dunlap RE, Gallup GH, Gallup AM. Of Global Concern: Results of the Health of the Planet Survey. *Environment* 1993; 35(9):7–15, 33–40.

87. Stedman RC, Davidson DJ, Wellstead A. Risk and Climate Change: Perceptions of Key Policy Actors in Canada. *Risk Analysis* 2004; 24(4):1395–1406.

88. Flynn J, Slovic P, Mertz CK. Gender, Race, and Perception of Environmental Health Risks. *Risk Analysis* 1994; 15(6):1101–1108.

89. Johnson CY, Bowker JM, Cordell HK. Ethnic Variation in Environmental Belief and Behavior: An Examination of the New Ecological Paradigm in a Social Psychological Context. *Environment and Behavior* 2004; 36:157–186.

90. Parker JD, McDonough MH. Environmentalism of African Americans: An Analysis of the Subculture and Barriers Theories. *Environment and Behavior* 1999; 31:155–177.

91. Biel A, Nilsson A. Religious Values and Environmental Concern: Harmony and Detachment. *Social Science Quarterly* 2005; 86(1):178–191.

92. Schultz PW, Zelezny L, Dalrymple NJ. A Multinational Perspective on the Relation between Judeo-Christian Religious Beliefs and Attitudes of Environmental Concern. *Environment and Behavior* 2000; 32(4):576–591.

93. Sherkat DE, Ellison CG. Structuring the Religion-Environment Connection: Identifying Religious Influences on Environmental Concern and Activism. *Journal for the Scientific Study of Religion* 2007; 46(1):71–85.

94. McCright AM, Dunlap RE. Defeating Kyoto: The Conservative Movement's Impact on U.S. Climate Change Policy. *Social Problems* 2003; 50(3):348–373.

95. McCright AM, Dunlap RE. Challenging Global Warming as a Social Problem: An Analysis of the Conservative Movement's Counter-Claims. *Social Problems* 2000; 47(4):499–522.

96. Nilsson A, von Borgstede C, Biel A. Willingness to Accept Climate Change Strategies: The Effect of Values and Norms. *Journal of Environmental Psychology* 2004; 24(3):267–277.

97. Shearman D. Time and Tide Wait for No Man. *British Medical Journal* 2002; 325:1466–1468.

98. Gärling T, Schuitema G. Travel Demand Management Targeting Reduced Private Car Use: Effectiveness, Public Acceptability and Political Feasibility. *Journal of Social Issues* 2007; 63(1):139–153.

99. Tanner C. Constraints on Environmental Behaviour. *Journal of Environmental Psychology* 1999; 19:145–157.

100. Abrahamse W, Steg L, Vlek C, Rothengatter T. A Review of Intervention Studies Aimed at Household Energy Conservation. *Journal of Environmental Psychology* 2005; 25(3):273–291.

101. Steg L, Dreijerink L, Abrahamse W. Why are Energy Policies Acceptable and Effective? *Environment and Behavior* 2006; 38(1):92–111.

102. Rothman DS. Measuring Environmental Values and Environmental Impacts: Going from the Local to the Global. *Climatic Change* 2000; 44:351–376.

103. Poortinga W, Pidgeon NF. Exploring the Dimensionality of Trust in Risk Regulation. *Risk Analysis* 2003; 23(5):961–972.

104. Tyler TR, Degoey P. Collective Restraint in Social Dilemmas: Procedural Justice and Social Identification Effects on Support for Authorities. *Journal of Personality and Social Psychology* 1995; 69(3):482–497.

105. Moser SC. In the Long Shadows of Inaction: The Quiet Building of a Climate Protection Movement in the United States. *Global Environmental Politics* 2007; 7(2):124–144.

106. Corral-Verdugo V, Frías-Armenta M. Personal Normative Beliefs, Antisocial Behavior, and Residential Water Conservation. *Environment and Behavior* 2006; 38(3):406–421.

107. Peterson TD, Rose AZ. Reducing Conflicts between Climate Policy and Energy Policy in the U.S.: The Important Role of the States. *Energy Policy* 2006; 34:619–631.

108. Vasi IB. Organizational Environments, Framing Processes, and the Diffusion of the Program to Address Global Climate Change among Local Governments in the United States. *Sociological Forum* 2006; 21(3):439–466.

109. O'Connor RE, Bord RJ, Fisher A. Rating Threat Mitigators: Faith in Experts, Governments and Individuals Themselves to Create a Safer World. *Risk Analysis* 1998; 18(5):547–556.

110. Lorenzoni I, Pidgeon NF, O'Connor RE. Dangerous Climate Change: The Role for Risk Research. *Risk Analysis* 2005; 25(6):1387–1398.

111. Melnick DJ, Navarro YK, McNeely J, Schmidt-Traub G, Sears RR. The Millennium Project: The Positive Health Implications of Improved Environmental Sustainability. *The Lancet* 2005; 365(946):723–725.

112. Oppenheimer M, Todorov A. Global Warming: The Psychology of Long Term Risk. *Climatic Change* 2006; 77:1–6.

113. Berkhout F, Hertin J, Gann DM. Learning to Adapt: Organisational Adaptation to Climate Change Impacts. *Climatic Change* 2006; 78:135–156.

114. Boiral O. Global Warming: Should Companies Adopt a Proactive Strategy? *Long Range Planning* 2006; 39:315–330.

115. Siebenhuner B, Carl-von-Ossietsky MA. Organizational Learning to Manage Sustainable Development. *Business Strategy and the Environment* 2007; 16:339–353.

116. Padula A. Inescapable Questions: Academia, Global warming, and the Energy Crisis. *Journal of Progressive Human Services* 2005; 16:1–4.

117. Uzzell D. Education for Environmental Action in the Community: New Roles and Relationships. *Cambridge Journal of Education* 1999; 29(3):397–413.

118. Zint MT. Advancing Environmental Risk Education. *Risk Analysis* 2001; 21(3):417–426.

119. Pooley JA, O'Connor M. Environmental Education and Attitudes: Emotions and Beliefs are What is Needed. *Environment and Behavior* 2000; 32(5):711–723.

120. Pruneau D, Doyon A, Langis J, Vasseur L, Ouellet E, McLaughlin E, et al. When Teachers Adopt Environmental Behaviors in the Aim of Protecting the Climate. *The Journal of Environmental Education* 2006; 37(3):3–12.

121. Smith J. Dangerous News: Media Decision Making about Climate Change Risk. *Risk Analysis* 2005; 25(6):1471–1482.

122. Daamen DDL, Staats H, Wilke HAM, Engelen M. Improving Environmental Behavior in Companies: The Effectiveness of Tailored Versus Nontailored Interventions. *Environment and Behavior* 2001; 33(2):229–248.

123. McComas K, Shanahan J. Telling Stories about Global Climate Change: Measuring the Impact of Narratives on Issue Cycles. *Communication Research* 1999; 26(1):30–57.

124. Li Z. 2007. Media Performance and Global Policy Making: A Comparative Study of Press Coverage on Global Warming. PhD diss., University of Pennsylvania.

125. Johnson BB, Chess C. From the Inside Out: Environmental Agency Views About Communications with the Public. *Risk Analysis* 2006; 26:1395–1407.

126. Antilla L. Climate of Scepticism: US Newspaper Coverage of the Science of Climate Change. *Global Environmental Change Part A*, 2005 12; 15(4):338–352.

127. Palfreman J. A Tale of Two Fears: Exploring Media Descriptions of Nuclear Power and Global Warming. *Review of Policy Research* 2006; 23(1):23–43.

128. Viscusi WK, Chesson H. Hopes and Fears: The Conflicting Effects of Risk Ambiguity. *Theory and Decision* 1999; 47(2):153–178.

129. Ereaut G, Segnit N. *Warm Words: How Are We Telling the Climate Story and Can We Tell It Better?* London: Institute for Public Policy Research. 2006.

130. Chess C, Johnson BB, Gibson G. Communicating about Environmental Indicators. *Journal of Risk Research* 2005; 8(1):63–75.

131. Trettin L, Musham C. Is Trust a Realistic Goal of Environmental Risk Communication? *Environment and Behavior* 2000; 32(3):410–426.

132. Olli E, Grendstad G, Wollebaek D. Correlates of Environmental Behaviors: Bringing Back Social Context. *Environment and Behavior* 2001; 33:181–208.

133. Pol E, Castrechini A. City-Identity-Sustainability Research Network: Final words. *Environment and Behavior* 2002; 34(1):150–160.

134. Lubell M. Environmental Activism as Collective Action. *Environment and Behavior* 2002; 34(4):431–454.

135. Pol E. The Theoretical Background of the City-Identity-Sustainability Network. *Environment and Behavior* 2002; 34(1):8–25.

136. Vorkinn M, Riese H. Environmental Concern in a Local Context: The Significance of Place Attachment. *Environment and Behavior* 2001; 33(2):249–263.

137. Wester-Herber M. Underlying Concerns in Land-Use Conflicts: The Role of Place Identity in Risk Perception. *Environmental Science & Policy* 2004; 7:109–116.

138. Uzzell D, Pol E, Badenas D. Place Identification, Social Cohesion, and Environmental Sustainability. *Environment and Behavior* 2002; 34(1):26–53.

139. Evans GW, Saltzman H, Cooperman JL. Housing Quality and Children's Socioemotional Health. *Environment and Behavior* 2001; 33(3):389–399.

140. Brandon G, Lewis A. Reducing Household Energy Consumption: A Qualitative and Quantitative Field Study. *Journal of Environmental Psychology* 1999; 19(1):75–85.

141. Osbaldiston R, Sheldon KM. Promoting Internalized Motivation for Environmentally Responsible Behavior: A Prospective Study of Environmental Goals. *Journal of Environmental Psychology* 2003; 23(4):349–357.

142. Albrecht SM. Forging New Directions in Science and Environmental Politics and Policy: How Can Co-operation, Deliberation and Decision Be Brought Together? *Environment, Development and Sustainability* 2001; 3:323–341.

143. Schofer E, Hironaka A. The Effects of World Society on Environmental Protection Outcomes. *Social Forces* 2005; 84(1):25–47.

# Index